W9-CET-862

THE CAREGIVER'S GUIDE TO DEMENTIA

THE CAREGIVER'S GUIDE TO

Dementia

Practical Advice for Caring

for Yourself and Your Loved One

Gail Weatherill, RN, CAEd

ROCKRIDGE
PRESS

For general information on our other products and services or to obtain technical support, please contact our Customer Care Department within the United States at (866) 744-2665 or outside the United States at (510) 253-0500.

Rockridge Press publishes its books in a variety of electronic and print formats. Some content that appears in print may not be available in electronic books and vice versa.

TRADEMARKS: Rockridge Press and the Rockridge Press logo are trademarks or registered trademarks of Callisto Media Inc. and/or its affiliates in the United States and other countries, and may not be used without written permission. All other trademarks are the property of their respective owners. Rockridge Press is not associated with any product or vendor mentioned in this book.

Interior and Cover Designer: Richard Tapp
Art Producer: Michael Hardgrove
Editor: Seth Schwartz
Production Manager: Riley Hoffman
Production Editor: Melissa Edeburn

ISBN: Print 978-1-64611-392-7 | Ebook 978-1-64611-393-4
R0

FOR EACH ONE
that I have loved and lost:
Mommy, Nanny, Beautiful
Mary, Crazy Roger, Miss Ray,
Dr. T, and "Boss"; you are my
great cloud of witnesses.

Contents

Introduction   ix

PART ONE: **UNDERSTANDING DEMENTIA**

Chapter One: Dementia Explained 3

Chapter Two: A Caregiver's Journey Begins 21

PART TWO: **CARING FOR SOMEONE WITH DEMENTIA**

Chapter Three: Common Behavioral and Mood Changes 35

Chapter Four: Common Daily Living Changes 63

Chapter Five: Financial and Legal Decisions 89

Chapter Six: End-of-Life Care 111

PART THREE: **CARING FOR YOURSELF**

Chapter Seven: How Caregiving Affects You 125

Chapter Eight: Work–Life Balance 137

Chapter Nine: Staying Healthy and Resilient 145

Resources 160
References   164
Index   169

Introduction

If you're a dementia caregiver, kudos to you for picking up this book. I'm glad you're here. For a long time, I've worked with people with dementia and their caregivers. I love to show them that the glass is half full, that there are many days and moments of sheer joy yet to be lived.

Within these pages, you will find a broad picture of dementia caregiving. We're going to look at the illnesses that cause dementia and their treatment. We'll go over the most common changes for people living with dementia and how you can provide the best support. Your mental stability is the single most critical factor in your loved one's quality of life. So, we will talk about your own wellness—a lot.

For each subject, I provide bulleted lists of actions you can take to improve your health and your caregiving. You'll find things you can do, things to say to and ask your loved one, and things to say to and ask doctors and other health care professionals, lawyers, accountants, therapists, and friends.

My hope is that you'll feel a little better prepared to face a new reality with the person you take care of. I'll provide resources you can use in the future and remind you that you have options even when it feels like you don't.

As a registered nurse for 40 years, I've cared for hundreds of people living with dementia and their families. Specializing in this care meant becoming a certified Alzheimer educator.

I've also served as the director of nursing in a long-term nursing home and assisted-living facility. I cofounded an online support group that has grown to 50,000 caregivers in more than 100 countries. The work is in my blood.

If I've learned anything in my years of caregiving for people with dementia, it's that we are not just our brains. Thought and language may come from the brain, but they're not the whole story of who we are. We are sentient beings. We have a soul that's not subject to physical disease.

When the day comes that you feel like your loved one is gone, remember their soul. Remember their values. Remember their priorities in life. Remember the feelings the two of you shared.

None of those things can be destroyed by dementia. They exist independent of space and time. Hold on to them.

Know that no matter how far away your loved one seems to be, they're still here. They feel you. They know you're here. They know you're doing all you can do.

Maybe they can't tell you how they feel in the ways they used to, but dementia cannot erase your loved one. They're in there, and they love you. Nothing will ever change that.

I send you best wishes on your caregiving journey. You have my utmost respect. Hold tight to the person your loved one still is. And never doubt that what the brain cannot remember, the heart cannot forget.

PART ONE

UNDERSTANDING DEMENTIA

CHAPTER ONE

DEMENTIA EXPLAINED

BOB

Bob was a retired engineer with a PhD in thermal engineering from Stanford University. He'd worked on the California governor's commission on alternative energy sources. Retirement felt anticlimactic to him. But his wife, Gloria, was holding him to his promise of traveling while they were still young.

A few months into Bob's retirement, Gloria started noticing the odd comment from him here and there. One day, Bob had to call AAA because he'd run out of gas on Route 15. He had always kept his car immaculate and the tank topped up for every occasion. Then came the notices that their checking account was overdrawn. A sharp businessman like Bob didn't let this kind of thing happen.

The day Bob headed out to pick up milk and ended up at a Walmart two towns over was the day Gloria put her foot down. Something wasn't right, and he was going to see a doctor whether he wanted to or not. Bob agreed, to keep the peace, but inwardly he worried.

What if something really was wrong? What if these incidents were the result of more than the normal strain of adjusting to retired life? Gloria waited for that first appointment with her own sense of dread. All the while, she hoped she was making a mountain out of a molehill.

Dementia Defined

Dementia is not a disease. *Dementia* is a broad term for symptoms caused by brain disease. It's a loss of cognitive functioning.

Cognition is our ability to think, to remember, and to reason. Dementia shows up most often as memory loss. But brain disease can affect many areas of the brain, resulting in many other symptoms.

Dementia can cause difficulty controlling one's emotions or trouble with finding words. It can present as personality changes or an inability to focus or pay attention. Struggles with reasoning, thinking straight, or remembering things are hallmarks of dementia.

The loss of cognitive functioning results in unusual behaviors. When we see these behaviors, there's trouble in the person's thinking, remembering, and/or reasoning. A problem in these functions means disease is affecting the brain. This process is a part of brain failure.

Brain failure is a term we don't often hear when talking about dementia, but brain failure is what we're facing. Everyone has heard of heart failure. Most have heard of kidney failure. When the conditions of body systems cause an organ to not do its job properly, *failure* is the term used because the organ is now *failing* in its function in the body. The same thing can happen to the brain.

Dementia is a result of brain failure. When the heart fails, it can't properly pump blood to all parts of the body. When kidneys fail, they can't filter out toxins and excess fluid as blood passes through them. When the brain fails, it can't think straight, remember, or reason. A person with dementia is experiencing brain failure.

WHEN IT'S NOT DEMENTIA

Given all the myths about dementia, it's worth talking about what dementia is not. Mental health difficulties, like depression or an anxiety disorder, can mimic dementia. Testing anyone with dementia symptoms should include ruling out such conditions.

Mild cognitive impairment (MCI) is a diagnosis often surrounded by misunderstanding. Many think MCI is early Alzheimer's disease (AD). This assumption is not correct. MCI involves symptoms that go beyond the normal changes of aging. Their effects center on memory, language, and judgment. The symptoms stop short of what would be classified as dementia.

The difference between MCI and AD is in the severity of symptoms. In MCI, symptoms can be annoying but don't interfere with normal activities in life. With AD, dysfunctional memory, thinking, and reasoning cause greater disruption of daily life.

MCI does not always progress to AD. Studies show that 15 percent of those with MCI develop AD. The MCI glass is more than half full, considering that 8 out of 10 people with the condition don't get worse. Some may even get better over time. The reasons aren't fully understood.

Delirium is another symptom sometimes confused with dementia. Unlike dementia, delirium comes on rapidly. An acute medical problem, like infection, brain injury, or metabolic imbalance, can cause delirium. Surgery can also lead to sudden onset of delirium. Delirium may become permanent if untreated, so be sure to seek medical advice if your loved one has a rapid, marked decline in cognitive function.

An acute medical problem is one that occurs within a short period. People rarely decline overnight from dementia. An infection (such as urinary tract infection, which we'll talk about in chapter 4) is a much more likely culprit. Delirium comes on fast; dementia develops gradually.

Delirium manifests as severe confusion and rapid changes in functional abilities. Hallucinations or hyperactivity is often present. I often see delirium in older people during hospital stays. A person sick enough to need hospital care is sick enough to experience delirium.

The good news about delirium is that it generally goes away as the acute illness is treated. Delirium is not dementia. But a person with dementia is likely to experience delirium with any acute illness. We should think of delirium when someone with dementia has a sudden decline in function.

ASSESSING SYMPTOMS

Some conditions that cause the symptoms of dementia are reversible. The first step in a dementia assessment should be to rule out reversible causes. Ruling out conditions one by one can take a long time. But the time and effort are worth it on the off chance that the problem is something fixable.

Reversible causes of dementia symptoms include infection, vitamin deficiency, and thyroid dysfunction. Medication issues can be at fault especially in people taking multiple medications. Dementia due to excess fluid in the brain may resolve with a shunt or drain placement.

Brain tumors are another cause of dementia symptoms that may be treatable. Singer Kris Kristofferson lived three years diagnosed with Alzheimer's. A doctor then discovered he had Lyme disease. With appropriate treatment, his symptoms disappeared. Looking for the causes of dementia means leaving no stone unturned.

A critical point to understand is that dementia is not a normal part of aging. Advancing age is a risk factor for dementia but doesn't invariably lead to it. The following table distinguishes changes that are a normal part of aging from signs of dementia.

NORMAL CHANGE OR A SIGN OF DEMENTIA?

NORMAL AGING CHANGE	SIGN OF DEMENTIA
Entering a room and forgetting why you went there	Getting lost in a familiar place
Forgetting a new acquaintance's name	Forgetting the name of a close friend or family member
Misplacing items occasionally, but later finding them	Putting things in unusual places, like placing keys in the freezer
Forgetting something you were told	Asking the same questions over and over again, like "Where is my car?"
Making a bad decision now and then	Making frequent poor choices or exhibiting unusual risk-taking
Experiencing vision changes resulting in misty or cloudy eyesight	Having trouble judging distances or knowing if an object is moving or still, or seeing things others don't see

Types of Dementia

There are many diseases that cause brain failure resulting in dementia. Each disease has its own mechanism for damaging brain cells. Each has certain patterns—where it starts in the brain and which brain regions it affects most often. Diseases also vary in how they affect people's rate of decline as each disease progresses.

In this section, you'll find descriptions of the primary diseases that cause dementia. Their order reflects their prevalence in the United States. We begin with a look at the most common dementias, followed by rarer forms.

A word of warning: There's *a lot* of information in the next few pages. If you're human (and I'm assuming you are), there are a thousand thoughts and fears swirling in your mind right now. Give your brain a break as you read on.

In this case, being kind to yourself means not trying to digest all these diseases and facts at once. The last thing you need is to worry about every single type of dementia and whether it's what you're facing. Armchair diagnosing is best left to football fans.

ALZHEIMER'S DISEASE

AD is the most common cause of dementia, affecting 60 to 80 percent of people with dementia. The disease results from the buildup of certain proteins (amyloid and tau) in the brain.

These abnormal deposits of amyloid and tau form into plaques and tangles. You can think of amyloid plaques as blobs and tau tangles as strings of protein. Either form prevents brain cells from functioning as they should, leading to dementia.

Memory loss is often the primary symptom of AD, which is thought to start in the hippocampus, the brain region controlling most of memory. Other symptoms seen in AD include trouble finding words, irritability, and confusion.

As millions live with AD and millions more develop it, the race is on to find how AD starts and how to block that process. With more cells in the human brain than stars in the galaxy, this puzzle has long escaped a solution.

For now, there are few medical treatment options. These options do not cure; they might slow the rate of progression. Like most brain diseases causing dementia, AD is currently incurable.

The usual course of treatment is to start with donepezil (Aricept). The doctor will then add memantine (Namenda) a few months later. If both drugs are started at the same time, it's hard to tell which one causes any side effects that come up. Stomach or intestinal problems are the most common side effects.

Despite research efforts, there have been no new medical treatments for AD since 2003. This fact alone illustrates the complexity of finding a cure. Until something changes, prevention remains our best hope.

Measures we take for heart health are the same we should take for brain health. These measures include controlling high blood pressure, keeping a healthy weight, and exercising regularly.

On average, people with AD live 3 to 11 years beyond diagnosis. Some people do not survive that long, whereas others live up to 20 years after a diagnosis. With brain failure due to dementia, we never know how much time remains.

VASCULAR DEMENTIA

Vascular dementia differs from other forms of dementia in its mechanism. Vascular dementia is not a degenerative disease. It results from impaired blood flow to brain cells due to changes in the blood vessels that feed the brain. Brain cells are greedy little buggers. When their supply of oxygen and other critical elements fails, cells die in a short period of time.

Blood flow to the brain slows or stops when there are blockages from plaque in the vessels or breaks in the vessels. If the interruption in flow lasts or is widespread, a person can experience a stroke. However, cell death short of a full-blown stroke occurs much more often and can cause dementia.

A blood flow blockage may be temporary. The plaque blocking flow can loosen from the blood vessel wall to float to a larger blood vessel, which would allow blood flow to start again. This occurrence accounts for some of the day-to-day changes in a person's dementia symptoms. Mini-strokes, or transient ischemic attacks, result from temporary blockages that open again.

When brain blood vessels leak or develop a tear, blood escapes into the tissues. The brain sits in the cramped space inside the skull. As the buildup of blood grows, there's nowhere for the brain to go. Pressure increases inside the brain, which impairs or kills cells. Brain failure with dementia results when enough cells die or malfunction.

Any chronic health condition that causes blood vessel damage can cause vascular dementia. The biggest offenders are high blood pressure and uncontrolled diabetes. Preventing or treating vascular dementia hinges on controlling these conditions. Doctors may recommend blood thinners for some patients to prevent clots in the brain.

Vascular dementia can originate anywhere in the brain. For this reason, the symptoms vary depending on the affected region. These variations in location also make the course of vascular dementia difficult to predict.

LEWY BODY DEMENTIA

Lewy body dementia (LBD) is another type of dementia. A Lewy body is a clump of a protein called alpha-synuclein. Lewy bodies develop for unknown reasons. Their effect depends on where they form in the brain.

LBD often starts with movement difficulties. Muscle rigidity, tremors, and a shuffling walk are common. The affected person is likely to receive a diagnosis of Parkinson's disease. As time passes, more distinctive symptoms rule out a simple Parkinson's diagnosis.

Symptoms of LBD are unique from other types of dementia. They include visual hallucinations, sleep disorders, and difficulty carrying out mental tasks. Memory tends to be minimally affected.

Sleep disorders in LBD are often severe. REM sleep disorder causes bizarre behaviors during sleep that seem as if a person is acting out their dreams. They may talk in their sleep, experience sudden violent movements, or fall out of bed. These sleep symptoms often occur years before other symptoms do.

Dementia with Lewy bodies often affects the autonomic nervous system. This system controls blood pressure, heart rate, sweating, and digestion. Dysfunction causes dizziness and bowel issues, like chronic constipation.

When blood pressure bottoms out as a result of LBD, the person can experience a momentary blackout, which can lead to falls. Due to the blackout, the person remembers nothing about the cause of the fall.

As with most forms of dementia, there are no treatments to reverse or slow LBD. Medical treatment aims to control symptoms, but several medications have the opposite effect of their purpose. Many with the disease cannot take a wide range of medications for this reason.

Giving a person with LBD anti-Parkinson's medications often causes a worsening of behavioral symptoms. Antipsychotic medications intended to calm can create severe agitation and aggression. Giving *any* medication to someone with LBD warrants careful selection and monitoring.

Life expectancy for someone with LBD is difficult to predict. Averages run from 2 to 12 years following diagnosis. The younger the person is at the time of diagnosis, the faster the disease is likely to progress. It also tends to progress more quickly in women than in men.

MIXED DEMENTIA

With mixed dementia, a person has more than one of the brain diseases that cause dementia. VD and AD are the most common combination in mixed dementia. Most people with dementia past the age of 80 have this combination. With mixed dementia, it's hard to know how much each disease causes the person's symptoms. Medical treatment for each individual disease is the general standard.

FRONTOTEMPORAL DEMENTIA

Frontotemporal dementia (FTD) develops when the frontal and temporal lobes of the brain shrink because of cell damage by the protein tau or by another protein called TDP-43. These proteins can have a special affinity for the frontal and temporal lobes.

Their accumulation in those regions leads to FTD, or Pick's disease, as it was once called.

Symptoms reflect dysfunction of the frontal and temporal lobes. These lobes control executive function—what we use to make plans, solve problems, and make decisions. As FTD progresses, the ability to do these things declines. Impaired functions include mood regulation, emotional control, and inhibition.

FTD rarely causes memory problems, but behavioral symptoms can abound. Wide mood swings and a total lack of empathy are common. The lack of empathy can be especially brutal to others. In someone who previously was loving and supportive, this change can be devastating.

Disinhibition can result in odd behaviors and salty language unlike a person's lifelong norms. Sleep disturbances can eventually become a deal breaker for remaining in the home. Caregivers cannot run on little to no sleep forever. Episodes of anger and suspicion can lead to the threat of physical violence from some. This danger can become another motivation for seeking full-time care.

No medications have proven effective for the underlying brain disease of FTD. Memantine (Namenda) has helped a tiny number of people with FTD, but studies show it does not help most of the time. Treatment focuses on controlling the difficult symptoms FTD causes.

PARKINSON'S DISEASE DEMENTIA

Parkinson's disease dementia is the twin of dementia with Lewy bodies. Both diseases affect brain cells through the presence of Lewy bodies, and their symptoms mirror one another. Experts disagree on whether Parkinson's dementia and LBD are two separate diseases.

A diagnosis of Parkinson's dementia hinges on the individual's history of Parkinson's. If dementia develops at least one year after Parkinson's disease is diagnosed, it's called Parkinson's dementia. LBD develops within the first year of Parkinson's-like symptoms.

In Parkinson's disease dementia and LBD, unusual physical symptoms occur, such as visual hallucinations, shouting or thrashing about during sleep, and loss of facial expressions. Symptoms often get worse with drugs that would help in other dementias. The two types of dementia are treated similarly.

CREUTZFELDT-JAKOB DISEASE

Creutzfeldt-Jakob disease (CJD) is a rare brain disease that causes dementia. The National Institutes of Health report around 350 cases a year in the United States.

The vast majority of cases develop with no known origin. These cases are called *sporadic* CJD. Ten to 15 percent of those affected carry a rare genetic mutation that can pass from parent to child. Anyone with genetic CJD should seek genetic counseling to understand these risks.

The rarest cause of CJD is contamination from infectious sources, which is responsible for one in every million cases. Because infected beef has been a source of infection, CJD is associated with mad cow disease in the public's mind.

The primary trait of CJD is its rapid progression. The average life expectancy from the time of diagnosis is one year. There is no cure. Medical treatment focuses on symptom control and comfort care.

NORMAL PRESSURE HYDROCEPHALUS

Normal pressure hydrocephalus (NPH) comes from a buildup of excess fluid in the brain. This buildup rarely results from infections or tumors. Most of the time, there is no identifiable cause. NPH usually develops in people in their sixties and seventies.

The excessive fluid that characterizes NPH pushes on surrounding brain tissues, which causes mechanical damage and dementia. The cognitive symptoms may be mild and mistaken for other illnesses. Other symptoms of NPH are difficulty walking and loss of bladder control.If a person with NPH can tolerate surgery, they may opt for placement of a shunt in the brain. A shunt is a small tube that weaves from the brain to the abdomen so fluid can drain from the small, limited space within the brain to the large pool of abdominal fluid.

Studies show that shunt placement usually corrects walking difficulties. Cognitive decline and loss of bladder control tend to persist after surgery, but shunt placement may prevent further decline. Shunt placement is a common procedure that has risks but is deemed relatively safe.

HUNTINGTON'S DISEASE

Huntington's disease (HD) is a rare brain disease caused by a genetic mutation. The responsible gene can pass from parent to child. If a person has the gene, they will develop HD. Symptoms usually appear when the affected person is in their thirties or forties.

The progressive symptoms of HD fall into three categories: movement disturbances, dementia, and psychiatric disorders.

HD leads to extreme mobility and behavior problems that usually require 24-hour professional care. Life expectancy is 10 to 30 years from diagnosis.

When a person has the gene that causes HD, genetic counseling helps in family planning. Children have a 50-50 chance of inheriting the gene from an affected parent. If a child doesn't inherit the gene, the child's descendants are unlikely to experience HD.

WERNICKE-KORSAKOFF SYNDROME

Wernicke-Korsakoff syndrome (WKS) results from a thiamine deficiency. Thiamine is vitamin B_1, a critical nutrient in brain function. Thiamine deficiency can result from malnutrition, eating disorders, and chemotherapy. The most common cause is alcoholism, but stomach surgery, cancer, and overall malnutrition can also lead to its development.

Without early treatment, thiamine deficiency causes irreversible damage to brain cells. Restoring vitamin levels does not reverse the process. Symptoms of WKS include mental confusion, vision problems, and lack of muscle coordination.

Disorientation, memory impairment, and failure to form new memories are hallmarks of WKS. There is no cure for the disease. Medical management can only help control symptoms.

When WKS is due to alcoholism, the diagnosis is especially difficult for families. Years of alcohol abuse have likely created intense emotions within the family. The stigma associated with alcoholism carries over into dealing with WKS.

POSTERIOR CORTICAL ATROPHY

Posterior cortical atrophy (PCA) is a rare variation of AD. Its primary effects are visual and spatial. The posterior cortex of the brain interprets visual input. With PCA, the eyes may be taking in images with no trouble, but the brain isn't processing them accurately.

Most people with PCA attribute the problem to poor eyesight. They seek out ophthalmology care. But no change in an eyeglasses prescription is going to correct the brain's inability to interpret what it's seeing.

Symptoms of PCA include difficulty reading and judging distances. A person may be unable to tell if an object is moving or stationary. It may be unclear whether one or multiple objects are in sight. Some with PCA experience hallucinations.

PCA symptoms arise most often between the ages of 50 and 65. The disease is often missed during diagnosis and labeled as AD. There's no treatment to deter the progression of PCA.

Diagnosis and Next Steps

I hope that seeing the many causes of dementia helps you understand why it can take so long to get a diagnosis. Diagnosis often becomes a process of elimination that begins with ruling out the most common causes.

Most family physicians or geriatricians refer patients to a neurologist for a full dementia workup. Sometimes the patient or family must push for further testing. Don't be shy if you have concerns. The doctor knows less about how compromised an individual's function is than the affected person and their family do. You're the experts in what's happening daily.

A diagnostic workup leading to an accurate diagnosis requires more than one method of assessment. The more comprehensive the approach, the more likely the conclusions will be accurate.

The process starts with a detailed history and physical, including medical and family histories. It's important to look at the nature, frequency, and approximate start of symptoms. Blood work can be used to check for vitamin deficiencies and metabolic issues.

Radiologic imaging should also be included. I've seen someone with a brain tumor diagnosed with AD. A misdiagnosis can be reached when scans aren't included in the initial workup.

The most commonly ordered scan is magnetic resonance imaging, or MRI. An MRI can show infections, tumors, and vascular problems in the brain. It can also show levels of activity in each region of the brain. An MRI does not clearly show the plaques and tangles seen with AD.

The amyloid PET scan uses new technology to test for amyloid buildup in the brain. As a new test, it isn't covered by many insurance companies. Medicare has covered the scan only as part of a research study. This trend has been changing in recent years.

You should always ask your insurance carrier for its current coverage policy.

Another aspect in diagnosis is neurocognitive testing, which is typically a three- to five-hour session everyone dreads. A miniature version is administered in a doctor's office, the "draw a clock and remember these three things" drill. But why the arduous testing over hours?

Neurocognitive testing is intricately designed. It measures the function of the many regions of the brain. By knowing which regions show impaired function, we have a better idea of which disease may be to blame.

One of the biggest challenges for families can be getting the person with symptoms to go to a doctor. They may resist for many reasons. Some people avoid doctors on general principle. Others are afraid of what the outcome will be. And some truly don't recognize any problem.

When a loved one refuses a doctor visit for memory-related or behavioral symptoms, you can get creative. You may need to back off for a few weeks for calm to return. Then make an appointment for some other need, like an annual physical or a follow-up on health issues.

You'll become an expert on finding ways to give doctors information that would cause a ruckus if shared during the visit. One way is by writing down your specific observations and concerns and handing the list to the nurse before the visit starts. You can also drop it off in advance for the doctor to review.

Any diplomatic doctor will handle the visit without disclosing your communication. If they blow your cover without considering consequences, it could be time to doctor shop. If you're indeed facing a dementia diagnosis, you'll need a physician you can trust. More on that in chapter 2.

Another dilemma is when someone goes for cognitive testing but leaves early in a huff. Nobody wants to feel dumb, and being asked question after question that they can't answer can be humiliating.

If a loved one refuses to go to testing at the last minute or storms out after five minutes, don't worry. This behavior tells the clinician something about the person's current state. Extensive cognitive testing is helpful but not always critical for a diagnosis.

WHAT TO ASK YOUR DOCTOR

- Given the history of how my loved one's symptoms started, do you have any idea of what the diagnosis probably is?

- What kinds of tests are needed? Where are they given? Can I be there during the testing? How long does it usually take?

- What will the tests tell us? How long will it take to get the results?

- Should we be seeing a neurologist at this point, or is it too early to say?

How Are You Doing?

I'll ask you this question often. It's important. I will guide you from your early suspicions to wherever this journey takes you. I meant what I said. So, let's begin.

The thought of a loved one having a brain disease with dementia is enough to terrify anyone. Our personality, personal experiences, and relationship with the one who may be ill color our reactions. Trust me, if you even know your own name right now, you're doing well.

To survive this journey, you'll need to learn to gauge your own well-being—something few of us practice regularly. Your thoughts may be all over the place: *My life is over. This is too hard. I can't do this. I'm doing a rotten job.* Those thoughts drown us. My aim is to keep you afloat.

Here's what to do: Set aside 15 minutes to sit and be quiet. There are 1,440 minutes in a day; you can spare 15. Ask yourself the following questions. Write out the answers. This exercise would be a great time to use a journal or, my favorite, a spiral notebook from a dollar store. You'll be surprised how useful your notes may be one day. Ask yourself these questions:

- On a scale from 1 to 10, how afraid of the future am I right now?
- The best thing I did for my family this week was . . .
- The best thing I did for myself this week was . . .

Your other assignment for today? Breathe. You can do this. You're not alone.

CHAPTER TWO

A CAREGIVER'S JOURNEY BEGINS

SOFIA

"You have dementia. Probably Alzheimer's disease." Sofia looked from the doctor's face to her mother sitting across from him. It occurred to her that this feeling must be what people meant when they said it was like the air was sucked out of the room.

Sofia wondered why she felt so surprised. She had seen this coming for months now. But her mother had always been a master of social graces—on the phone and often in person, she'd covered for her lapses.

This woman was her beautiful mother. A woman she'd never seen leave the house without lipstick and matching accessories. The favorite hostess among her parents' crowd. The business office manager who could no longer follow simple mathematics.

Now, this doctor was announcing a disease that would change their lives. So matter-of-fact, as if the subject were heartburn. Sofia watched as he scrawled a prescription and handed it past her mother and into her own hands.

"Give her this once a day. It might help. If you have any questions, you can get answers from the Alzheimer's Association. Just go online." And just like that, the appointment was over. Sofia and her mother walked out in silence. They stopped to schedule a three-month follow-up. Sofia wondered what they would be following up on.

Would her mother be better? Or would she even know who Sofia was by then? In the span of a 15-minute doctor visit, the world had turned upside down.

Changing Relationships

We are social creatures. Our connections with other human beings affect our sense of self and what we live for. When dementia enters the picture, it can be an enormous threat to those connections. As roles shift, the emotional toll can loom large.

What adult child relishes becoming the parent to their father or mother? A sibling who has looked up to a big brother all her life may not know how to be the strong one. The husband of a beloved partner of many decades wonders how he could possibly become a caregiver.

Our experience with changing roles will hinge on our attitude about them. First, these changes rarely happen overnight. You'll likely have time to prepare for shifts. There will be moments when your awareness hits all at once, but the process itself is gradual.

Remember that getting a dementia diagnosis doesn't suddenly strike a person incompetent. The person who walked out of that doctor's office with you is the same person who walked in. The two of you are facing significant losses, but there's time to comfort each other before they happen.

If you're an adult child whose parent has always been a source of strength, it can feel like your moorings are gone. Some children worry about the future of their independence as roles change. Or maybe your parent was distant or even abusive long before dementia developed.

Spouses experience the most complicated role changes as dementia progresses. Is your spouse your best friend? It's hard when the person who helped make decisions, asked how your day was, and made you laugh can't do these things anymore.

For spouses, the changes of dementia can have a profound effect on sex and intimacy. We'll talk about this more in chapter 4, but it warrants mention here. Then there are the dreams of retirement that the two of you relished together. It's normal to grieve the life that you thought you would have.

Dementia caregivers come from all sorts of relationships. You may not be a relative. I once had a longtime client who never married and had no children. When dementia came calling, I eventually moved her into my home. The lack of a lifelong history can sometimes make such a decision much less complicated.

Roles of the primary caregiver and the person living with dementia aren't the only ones to change. Sharing a new diagnosis with friends and family will draw a variety of reactions. It's important for you and your loved one to decide whom, when, and what to tell.

The Alzheimer's Association has gathered the perspectives of many people living with dementia. One experience holds true across all groups: The reactions of others to the diagnosis are often worse than the disease itself. No one with dementia or their caregiver can escape this reality.

If your hair is as white as mine, you may recall when having cancer was shameful. A diagnosis certainly wasn't anything you talked about openly. It was common practice not to tell the ill person what was wrong.

Fast-forward to the 21st century. We talk about cancer like we talk about our diets. The stigma is almost completely gone. It moved next door to those affected by dementia. Now, there are many who refuse to say "the D word" to their loved one.

Hearing that a friend or family member has dementia evokes many emotions. Our own fear of a similar fate can easily overshadow the sadness for those we care about. We feel inadequate and wonder, *How am I supposed to handle this? What am I supposed to say? Will they even know who I am? Will they remember that they saw me, and we talked? What's the point?*

Family and friends who live close by but rarely engage can cause great pain. I hear the same stories over and over: The friend who faithfully called every Monday night, the minister who often visited during times of serious illness, the cousin who lives a mile away and frequently dropped by to say hello—before dementia they all entered your orbit. Then silence on all fronts.

Then there's the family doctor who turns away with helpless feelings of having nothing to offer. And more disappearing friends and family, with their cries of "I can't bear to see him like that." Do they think you're glad to be there in their place?

The withdrawal of those you need at the time you need them the most is one of the biggest sources of family conflict. Old rivalries and hurt feelings often resurface in full force.

It would be great if everyone set aside their differences and rallied in a time of crisis. But the movie *It's a Wonderful Life* isn't real life. Demanding something from someone who cannot give it is futile. We must look to others to support us. Our sanity depends on it.

Whether you're caring for a parent, a spouse, or someone else, dementia caregiving is a journey of fine lines. One is the line between recognizing reality and projecting future sadness onto today.

One silver lining of dementia entering our lives is how it teaches us to stay in the present. This lesson isn't an easy one. We're accustomed to looking ahead, planning, and, in many cases, worrying more than a little. Nothing escalates these habits quite like a dementia diagnosis.

In dementia caregiving, the tendency to worry about the future can become lethal. One in six spousal caregivers don't survive the journey; they die first. The physical toll of constant worry is much to blame.

We must harness our thoughts for both our own sake and the sake of our loved ones. If you go down, where does that leave them? Ask this question any time you're tempted to make caring for yourself a bottom-rung priority.

There are two main approaches that help during this period of changing roles: (1) recognizing and acknowledging changes as they occur and (2) allowing yourself to grieve what was and is no longer.

Few approaches to change cause more pain than clinging to old patterns. The more we insist on having what has been, the harder it becomes to see the joy in what remains. And the good news is that there is a great deal of joy yet to come your way.

WHAT TO DO

- Make a list of roles your loved one has played in your life. Make a list of roles you've played in theirs. Mark which ones are still intact.

- Write down some of the little things that happen that remind you that you're still you and your loved one is still your loved one. Recognizing a favorite song? Working in the garden? Pay attention to these small but significant moments.

- Allow yourself time and space to grieve the loss of former roles. Anticipatory grief is a real thing. Just don't park there for too long.

- Talk with someone you trust about your changing roles, such as a friend, spiritual advisor, close family member, or therapist.

- Make a list of tasks or gifts that someone could provide in lieu of being on the front lines of caregiving. For example, your sibling lives in California and you're in Maine. Could they take over Mom's finances and bill paying? Could they chip in for a home health aide to give you a break?

- Consider sending friends and family a heartfelt message up front. Tell them you know they may feel uncomfortable, but you and your loved one need and want them in your lives. Tell them things that your loved one still enjoys during visits. List some of the ways they can help so you can avoid the vague "Let me know if you need anything."

Working with a Dementia Care Team

Dementia caregiving is best tackled with a solid foundation of professional advisors. These advisors are key to your and your loved one's well-being. We are physical, mental, and spiritual beings. Both you and your loved one will need support in each of these areas.

DOCTORS

Cast your net wide when assembling a dementia care team. Physicians are often the first professionals you enlist, including a few specialists.

Family doctors often refer their patients to a neurologist for a dementia workup. Neurologists are doctors who focus on diagnosing and treating diseases of the nervous systems. Beyond making a diagnosis and prescribing indicated drugs, neurologists may have a limited role. Many neurologists know more about diseases than about symptom control.

In this situation, a geriatric psychiatrist can be a great solution. A good geriatric psychiatrist knows the brain and how drugs affect its function. Psychiatrists focus on behaviors and the impact on well-being in both patient and caregiver. They understand that trial and error is necessary for finding the best treatment.

Other health care disciplines in dementia care are nursing, social work, and various therapies. Nurses focus on physical and mental needs to see the big picture. Social workers can help navigate family dynamics and changing care needs. They also may help address insurance regulations, a nightmare for most of us.

Specialized therapists support the daily needs of those living with dementia. Their role is to maximize abilities and help people adjust to new challenges. These professionals can increase the quality of life for people with dementia.

Occupational therapists focus on the ordinary tasks of daily living—matters we take for granted until we forget how to do them. Think cooking, using the bathroom, or brushing your teeth.

Physical therapists can help a person maintain physical strength and function. Recreational therapists address the need for meaningful activity. Anyone living with dementia may benefit from the help of any or all of these practitioners.

We can't forget spiritual needs, our own and those of our loved one. Those with spiritual practices before dementia can find strength in continuing them. A trusted member of the clergy or a spiritual advisor can be enlisted for your team. They need to know their support matters to you and your loved one.

One more professional I recommend for any dementia care team is a psychotherapist or counselor, whether a licensed professional counselor, a clinical social worker, or a psychologist. Dementia caregiving is no ordinary bump in the road of life. Emotions run high and relationships are tested. There's no reason to handle it alone.

If your car started making weird noises every time you accelerated, you would seek professional advice. Your heart and soul are more important than your car. Studies show that the number one factor in the well-being of a person with dementia is the emotional stability of their primary caregiver. A professional counselor can help you.

Almost every major medical center today runs special programs for dementia patients. These programs can be a one-stop shop for all things dementia care. Comprehensive programs include medicine, nursing, social work, and various therapies. To find the nearest program, search online for "medical center dementia programs" in your area.

CLINICAL TRIALS

Clinical trials are another potential source of help. People enrolled in a clinical trial receive a high level of care at no cost to them, such as extra diagnostic testing, thorough assessment of their condition over time, and access to treatments not yet available to the public. Studies show enrollees do better than people at a similar stage of dementia who aren't in a trial. Participants have benefited even when the tested treatment didn't work. The extra care was the key.

Second, enrolling in a clinical trial means helping researchers find better treatments or even cures for dementia. Even if the results don't benefit your loved one directly, consider your children or your grandchildren. What would you do to spare them what you're going through?

The Alzheimer's Association keeps a current database called TrialMatch. The service isn't just for Alzheimer's studies. You can see where trials are conducted (some are online) and the qualifications for each study. You can find TrialMatch in the Resources section (page 160).

WHEN THINGS GO WRONG

Let's address the misadventures we all encounter in health care these days. We've all heard stories of arrogant, unhelpful doctors. We've seen overworked, defensive professionals concerned about saving their own necks. It may be called a health "care" system, but we don't always feel the care.

It's your right to choose the people you want on your caregiving team. You need every member to be someone you can count on to help. Life with dementia often lasts for years. Going the distance depends on the team supporting you.

If any professional produces more problems than solutions, it's not okay. You don't necessarily have to fire someone at the first sign of trouble. Discussing expectations up front and dealing with lapses as they occur are key.

This principle holds true for physicians and the home health aides coming in to give you a break. You'll encounter some who aren't there for you. Never be afraid to change horses midstream and find a new professional.

While I'm at it, here's another tip: The caregiver provides the best communication between specialists. Never assume that doctors, hospitals, facilities, or therapists share information or documents.

WHAT TO DO

Make a grab-and-go record about your loved one. Get a 1½-inch three-ring binder and a pack of at least five dividers.

- Label the dividers "Emergency Contacts," "Medical History," "Medications," "Professional Visits," and "Legal."

- In the first section, write down emergency contact names, relationships, addresses, phone numbers, and e-mail addresses. List them in the order of priority for contacting.

- In Medical History, record when your loved one was diagnosed with dementia and what tests were used to make the diagnosis. List any other medical conditions at play and any past surgeries. If your loved one has a do-not-resuscitate order, write that at the top of the page in big, bold letters.

- Also in Medical History, note the presence of metal by writing, "[Loved one's name] DOES [or DOES NOT] have metal in [his or her] body." Then list any metal plates, rods, artificial joints, valves, shrapnel, or pacemaker your loved one has.

- In the Medications section, write down the names of any medications along with the dose for each, the time(s) each drug is taken, and (if you know) when each medication began. If a doctor says to stop a medication, draw a single line through it. You should still be able to read what it was for future reference. Write the date of the change. Do the same thing if a dose is changed. Draw a line through the old dose, and write the new dose and the date of the change.

- Also in Medications, label a page "Allergies/Bad Reactions." List any known allergies, including what happens when your loved one takes that drug or food. If any medication has caused a bad reaction other than an allergy, specify the drug and what happened.

- Professional Visits should contain several pages of loose-leaf paper. Each time your loved one has any professional care encounter, record it here. This section is a good place to list questions you need to ask during visits and to take notes on the answers. Jot down any new plans during the visit. Include new prescriptions and medications to stop. Be sure to update your Medications section with these changes.

- Use the Legal section to keep a copy of any legal documents related to care (originals should be somewhere safer). These records should include do-not-resuscitate orders, power-of-attorney documents, and/or any advance directives, such as a living will.

It takes some time to put this record together. But I promise that having all this information in one place to carry with you will be worth every minute spent. You may want to include extra copies of the medical history and the medication list—it's safer than trusting someone who says, "I'll copy this and bring it back to you."

- What tests has my loved one had? What did they show?

- What medications will you start? What are they for? What side effects should I watch for? When should I call you if I'm worried about reactions to medications?

- How do you work with other specialists? Whom do I call for different problems?

- How often do you project seeing my loved one? What is the purpose of those visits?

- When will we talk about advance directives for my loved one?

How Are You Doing?

Navigating the changes in your relationship is one of the most challenging aspects of dementia caregiving. We've touched on some serious pain points in this chapter. How are you doing?

You may feel overwhelmed by the magnitude of your emotions, not to mention the twists and turns those emotions take in the course of any given day. If you bounce between rage, sorrow, and profound guilt, you are right on course.

If you waver between adoring your loved one and wanting to send them to the time-out corner for the rest of the day, you're 100 percent normal. There's no such thing as the perfect caregiver. You're going to do the best you can do. I promise you'll make mistakes, some little, some big. You'll get through them.

You don't have to be perfect. You do have to be there. Being there is way more than many family members are doing for their loved one.

As dementia caregivers, we must make a place for our emotions to go. If we don't, they'll cripple us. Here's an exercise to help.

Think of a friend you've cared about for a long time. Imagine they're facing the same caregiving situation you are. Take out a piece of paper and write them a note of encouragement.

When you finish, go back to the top. Strike through their name in the greeting, and substitute your name. Read aloud what you wrote to yourself. You deserve all the support and compassion you would offer to a friend living in your shoes.

PART TWO

CARING FOR SOMEONE WITH DEMENTIA

CHAPTER THREE

COMMON BEHAVIORAL AND MOOD CHANGES

BRENDA

Brenda sat down on the commode and prayed no one knew where she was. It had been eight months since her mother moved in with her and her family, eight months that felt like an eternity.

Brenda's mom, Dorothy, was 70 years old and had Alzheimer's. She'd managed to hide her troubles even though Brenda lived in town and visited often. Dorothy was smooth. Brenda had laughed at her mom's occasional "senior moments."

Then came the day a police officer called Brenda at work. It seemed Dorothy had started a small fire in her apartment building. She'd forgotten she'd put the kettle on for tea. Luckily, no one was hurt, but Dorothy's days of living alone were over.

Brenda's jaw dropped when Dorothy's doctor told her it had been a year since Dorothy came in complaining about her memory. He'd put her on Aricept and hadn't seen her since. Dorothy had always taken great pride in her independence, but Brenda never would have guessed her mom would with-hold this news.

A month later, a sulking Dorothy moved in with Brenda. Dorothy now had a daughter, a son-in-law, and two teenage grandchildren for company. There was plenty to do in the neighborhood—a park in walking distance and the pool during the summer. How could this new arrangement be a bad thing?

Bam! Brenda jumped a foot when she heard the front door slam. She scrambled to see what was going on. She reached the front door just in time to see Mom crossing the street in a hurry. Brenda turned and asked her son what happened.

"I don't know. One minute I was playing my music, and the next minute she was screaming at me to turn it off. You should do something about her, Mom. Grandma's making all of us crazy."

Anger and Aggression

Anger and aggression: the responses that strike fear in the hearts of dementia caregivers. Only about a third of people with dementia develop aggression. For those who do, it's the most common reason families are forced to place a loved one in a care facility.

Aggression is the verbal or physical result of anger gone unchecked. Humans get angry. Anger arises in response to perceived threats and unmet desires or expectations, or to hide emotions.

When our brains are on track, the frontal lobe regulates our emotions, preventing wide swings to one extreme or another. The frontal lobe works to keep us on an even keel.

The frontal lobe also inhibits impulsive actions. Throat-punching your boss or taking your pants off in an overheated restaurant seldom ends well. The frontal lobe tells us, "Don't do that."

Personality forms in the frontal lobe. Our level of tolerance for changing plans or unexpected outcomes is a part of our personality. We all know people who are easygoing. That trait is influenced by the frontal lobe.

When brain disease damages the frontal lobe, each of these functions falters. Anger easily slips into extremes of rage. No voice whispers, "Don't tell that lady she is fat." And any disruption of routine can cause profound distress.

Brain failure of this kind leads to what professionals call "catastrophic reactions," another way to say "losing it" in 21 letters. Either way, you know it when you see it.

Aggression may be verbal and can feel just as devastating as physical violence. Caregivers may be subject to all manner of verbal abuse. The saying that we always hurt the ones we love rings true in many households where dementia lives.

Violence, such as hitting, scratching, or biting, may erupt from the smallest stressor. Try telling an adult with dementia that they can no longer drive or have access to knives for cooking. These necessary precautions can lead to a firestorm.

Anger and aggression are no laughing matter for the dementia caregiver. The safety of both caregiver and care recipient may eventually require a professional care setting. Promises to never place a loved one in a home don't count when you're afraid to close your eyes at night.

There are things that we can do to reduce catastrophic reactions in our loved ones. Maintaining consistent routines, discovering triggers for aggression, and avoiding stressors can help. If your loved one has begun to display aggression, play detective. Learn what increases their stress level so you can step lightly around those triggers.

There are medications to reduce the frequency or severity of aggressive episodes. A practitioner may recommend antianxiety medications or prescribe a class of drugs called antipsychotics.

Antipsychotic drugs are controversial because of their potential side effects. On average, people taking antipsychotic drugs have a higher death rate than those who don't take them. A much more common side effect is oversedation. These drugs may affect balance, and falls may result.

Saying no to antipsychotic drugs, though, may be throwing out the baby with the bathwater. In 20 years of dementia nursing, I've seen these medications restore many people's quality of life. I've also seen them prevent the need to place a loved one in a care facility.

The key is vigilance when using any medication that acts on the brain. The brain's response to a drug is extremely individualized. You can give 10 people the same drug at the same dose and get 10 different reactions. Finding the right drug for the right person is often a process of trial and error.

Most horror stories about medications come from putting people on a drug without monitoring their response. In some care facilities, the goal is to keep people quiet. Oversedation is the result. As long as you're watchful for this side effect, using antipsychotic drugs may be a good option.

Geriatric psychiatrists tend to be the most skilled in prescribing medications for aggression. Neurologists who are knowledgeable in this area seem to be rare. If my loved one was showing difficult behaviors or moods, I'd hotfoot it to a geriatric psychiatrist.

QUESTIONS TO ASK ABOUT ALL MEDICATIONS

The best advice on any medication includes how it relates to the individual who will be taking it. Before taking or giving any medication to a loved one, ask the prescriber these questions.

- Are there medications that can help? If so, what are they?
- What are the side effects I should watch for with these medications?
- What time of day should I give them?
- How long does it take to know if the medication is helping?
- How long is it safe to be on this medication?
- How long do these medications actually help?

WHAT TO SAY

- When you see a loved one struggling, acknowledge how they may be feeling: "I'm sorry you feel so bad."

- Offer alternatives to frustrating tasks: "Let's go for a walk. You can work on that when we come back."

- After the storm has passed, reassure them. If they remember and regret anything they said or did, use phrases like "I know you didn't mean ..." Reminding a loved one of their words or actions will not change future behavior.

WHAT TO DO

- Avoid arguing. Brain failure can cause your loved one to think, see, or hear things that make no sense to you. You will *never* win an argument with a person with dementia.

- Keep instructions down to one step at a time. Skip the explanations; you'll lose your audience after the fourth word.

- Look for sources of your loved one's distress much like you would in response to a crying baby. Are they hungry, cold, in pain? Words may fail them, but all behavior has meaning.

- Pay attention to what was happening just before a meltdown. Was the room noisy? Were three people telling them what to do at the same time? Did they have to get up early for an appointment? Noise, confusion, and fatigue are common triggers.

- If your loved one becomes upset, make sure they're in a safe spot, then walk away. Give yourself and them a few minutes to cool down.

- As people with dementia lose language, they adapt by reading emotions in others. Keep a low, calm tone of voice. Use as few words as you can. Smile to give the idea of safety.

- Stick to a daily routine as much as possible. Any change in routine can cause confusion.

- Look for ways to insert exercise into their day. Burning off energy helps.

- Distract or redirect whenever you can. Move to a quieter room. Bring out a snack. Turn on their favorite music. If it didn't work on Monday, it may work on Wednesday.

- Go online and search for "geriatric psychiatrist" in your area. Even if you have to drive a ways to reach them, a good one is worth it.

- If you believe your loved one is a physical danger to self, you, or others, call 911. Always tell the dispatcher your loved one has dementia. Say they do not understand directions or what they are doing. This information will help first responders know the best approach.

WHAT TO ASK YOUR DOCTOR

Record some of your loved one's most difficult moments so you can show the doctor a quick video of what you're experiencing. (Ask a friend or family member to assist you with recording if you need help.) Without firsthand knowledge, it's hard to grasp how severe the symptoms can be. Video is your best demonstration tool for health care professionals and skeptical family members.

You may not want to describe details of the aggression to the doctor in front of your loved one. Make a list of the actions you're seeing. Include any patterns in time of day or circumstance and how often the episodes are happening. The list can be handed to the office nurse to give the doctor before the visit begins. I would write in big letters at the top, "PLEASE do not discuss details of these behaviors in front of my loved one."

- What do you think is the main cause of these aggressive episodes?

- How would you advise me to handle them? When should I contact you? When should I call 911?

- What would happen if my loved one had to be admitted to the hospital for aggression? Where would they be treated? What would that involve?

- See the "Questions to Ask About All Medications" sidebar earlier in this section (page 38) for additional questions.

Anxiety and Agitation

Anxiety is common in people with dementia. It causes many of their most difficult symptoms. To understand anxiety in dementia, we must understand its origins in all of us.

Anxiety is based in fear that our needs will not be met. Everyone needs security, physical and emotional comfort, meaningful activities, and relationships. We all desire dignity, privacy, and functional competence. These needs and desires are what makes us human.

When we're uncertain about how these needs will be met, we become anxious. This normal human response doesn't go away in the presence of brain failure. It only intensifies as confusion grows.

Imagine that one day you wake up in a remote, foreign village. People are talking, but you don't understand the words.

They don't understand you, either. You don't know what you're supposed to do or how you're going to get back home. You don't know when or how this ordeal will end.

Stressful? Of course. A normal response would be a level of anxiety that matches your circumstances. This experience is the world of a person living with dementia.

Your loved one's level of confusion will dictate their level of anxiety. The greater their confusion, the greater their anxiety is likely to be. Unfamiliar environments and circumstances increase anxiety. Your loved one attempts to understand the situation. When that fails, they become anxious.

A normal human response to anxiety is agitation. Agitation is a state of upset and disturbance in thinking. Agitation in a person with dementia shows up in many ways. These symptoms are some of the most difficult to deal with in dementia caregiving.

Restlessness, pacing, trying to leave; irritability and refusing to cooperate with any activity; crying and nonstop clinging to a familiar person—sound familiar? These states of agitation are often expressions of anxiety and needs that aren't being met.

For caregivers, it helps to see that these behaviors are attempts to fix a world turned upside down. Your loved one believes they won't be okay unless the situation is right-side up again. They're certain they must act now to avoid disaster.

In all of us, our human needs for safety, comfort, and relationships drive our behavior and desires. You might say these needs make up our humanity. And our humanity isn't subject to the ravages of brain disease.

Our loved one's humanity never leaves them, even when others forget that fact. No matter how baffling their anxiety symptoms become, they're acting out of need. Look beyond the symptoms to the human feelings that might be causing them. What we see is evidence that their humanity is still intact. They are *always* still in there somewhere.

WHAT TO SAY

- "I'm sorry you feel so bad. What bothers you the most?" Then zip your lip and let them talk. The idea is to give our loved one space to hold their feelings with them. We don't try to explain the sorrow away or cheer them up. Acknowledge the reality of the situation.

- "You're safe here." Changes in behavior are often rooted in fear. Reassuring them that all is well can help.

- "I'm here for as long as you need me. You're not alone." Give additional reassurance that your loved one is safe. You want them to know that you won't leave them to fend for themselves. Your loved one wants to hear the same things we all want to hear when we're anxious.

WHAT TO DO

- Use a calm, low-pitched tone of voice. People with dementia read your nonverbal cues much more than your words. Fewer words and warm reassurance are key.

- Minimize distractions in the environment, like the television or too many people around at one time.

- Try to put yourself in your loved one's shoes; imagine what distorted thoughts may be adding to their distress. Letting them talk things out can provide clues to the best way to help.

- Avoid explaining that their fears and anxiety are not based in reality. If Dad says there are aliens in the driveway, then there are aliens in the driveway, period. Better to ask what he thinks might make them leave than to tell him there's no such thing. Enter their reality. Well-intentioned attempts to help them see their fear is unfounded only make things worse.

- Attempt to distract or redirect. Ask for help with a task. Put on their favorite music. Share a snack.

- Diffusing essential oils, like lavender, can reduce anxiety. You can also put a tiny drop of lavender oil in a teaspoon of coconut oil or hand cream and rub it on your loved one's hands. When they begin to get upset, they can loosely cup their hands around their mouth and nose. Show them how to take slow, deep breaths to help relax.

- Keep to a daily routine. Predictability is a crucial deterrent to fear. Look for any patterns of increased anxiety at particular times of day or in particular circumstances.

- Keep them moving. The more physical activity they engage in, the less excess energy there is to invest in brooding.

- Consult your loved one's physician for advice on handling anxiety and agitation.

WHAT TO ASK YOUR DOCTOR

- How would you advise me to handle my loved one's anxiety?

- Are there steps we can take to avoid or minimize using medications for this behavior?

- What should I watch for as possible triggers for agitation and anxiety?

- See the "Questions to Ask About All Medications" sidebar (page 38) for additional questions.

Depression

"If you had dementia, you'd be depressed, too." I couldn't argue with the 52-year-old man sitting across from me. If you think the possibility of depression in someone with dementia means doctors routinely screen for it, think again. Underdiagnosis is rampant.

Diagnosing depression in someone with dementia is complicated, because the two illnesses share so many symptoms. Many of the symptoms of depression mimic symptoms of dementia. It becomes a puzzle of which came first.

There are some important differences between depression and dementia. Depression onset takes place over weeks to a few months rather than the years of dementia onset. People in early stages of dementia may feel ashamed, hopeless, or worthless following their diagnosis. These feelings are depression talking, not dementia.

Irritability, tearfulness, and appetite changes are common in depression. Social withdrawal and recurring thoughts of death or suicide are associated with depression. These symptoms are often more severe when due to depression than they would be with dementia alone.

I encourage all caregivers to request regular depression screenings for their loved one. If you notice signs or changes that may be depression, speak up. Ask that they be screened and treated if a diagnosis is confirmed. Treatment can help. You know your loved one; if you're concerned, you're probably right.

Treatment for depression may be medication based or not. The best results come from a combination of approaches. This scenario is another one where a geriatric psychiatrist is best equipped to recommend treatment. As with all medication use, there should be close monitoring for usefulness and side effects.

Here's a tip to help both depression and anxiety: If you can find mindfulness-based stress reduction (MBSR) training near you or online, take it. If your loved one is in the early stages of dementia, take them along with you. There's strong evidence that MBSR can benefit both caregiver and care recipient for years.

With MBSR, caregiver burden declines and the need for facility care can be delayed. Difficult behaviors are less frequent and severe. These benefits continue long after the one with dementia has forgotten the training. It's worth an online search.

WHAT TO SAY

- "I'm sorry you feel so bad. I know this feels like too much." Acknowledging your loved one's fears and sorrows is important. They want to know that you understand.

- "I'm here with you. I love you. We will go through this together. I won't leave you." A person with impaired cognition doesn't always understand that they're safe and that you won't leave them alone. You need to reassure them often.

- "I think there are some things we can do to help you feel better. I'll help find them." Everyone needs hope to survive. You can give your loved one hope that they won't always feel as bad as they do right now.

- "It's not okay that you feel this bad. We'll get help." Your loved one needs reassurance that their complaints are valid and that you'll help them get the care they need to feel better.

WHAT TO DO

- Trust your gut. If you think your loved one may be depressed, ask their doctor to assess them.

- Part of testing for depression is obtaining a history of symptoms. Before an office visit, jot down what you're seeing that makes you concerned. The doctor will ask when you first noticed these changes. Watch these symptoms to see if a treatment is helping.

- Many things that help anxiety also help depression. Strive for physical activity, such as walking, most days. Keep a daily routine. Get rest and sunshine. Lay off the junk food. Don't hide away from family or friends.

- Play your loved one's favorite music daily. Music is a proven antidote for depressive thoughts. Music with movement is even better. Get them off the sofa, turn off the TV, and shake a leg.

All these suggestions are easier said than done. Your loved one won't always buy into your efforts. No need to shovel another helping of guilt onto your plate. It's all trial and error, anyway. Try again tomorrow.

WHAT TO ASK YOUR DOCTOR

- Do you think these symptoms are caused by depression apart from the dementia?

- How can you tell?

- Are there signs I should always call you to report?

- See the "Questions to Ask About All Medications" sidebar (page 38) for additional questions.

Memory Loss and Confusion

Memory loss is the symptom most people associate with dementia. Confusion is memory loss's kid brother. Confusion in someone with dementia refers to being disoriented to time, place, or identity. The brain holds our memories, tells us who and where we are, and allows us to discern time. As brain disease progresses, these functions begin to falter and eventually fail completely.

In the early stages of dementia, memory loss and confusion tend to be mild. In some ways, this phase is the most painful leg of the journey. Our loved one has lost enough brain cells to be confused and forgetful. But they still have the brain power to know they don't know some things.

As brain failure progresses, confusion and memory loss grow. If a loved one says they've done the dishes for you, check the freezer. You wouldn't be the first to find dirty dishes "washed and put away" there. Correcting your loved one does nothing but upset and confuse them more.

It's often hard to fathom how profound their confusion can be. We want to explain. We want to convince. We might as well want to hit the lottery. The odds of success are about the same.

One of confusion's annoying traits is that it's seldom the same day to day. Has your loved one ever acted normally when company comes? Or kept it together for the five-minute phone call with your sibling, just long enough to convince said sibling that Mom is fine and you're neurotic?

It happens. Social graces can make it easy for people with dementia to fool us about how troubled they are. After holding themselves together for a while, our loved one will likely be exhausted and more confused than ever. Shopping, social occasions, and health appointments are draining. It can take days to fully recover from what used to be so easy.

Although confusion can vary day to day, a sudden increase can be a sign of trouble. Dementia almost never progresses from one level to the next overnight. Changes over a few days are usually due to some acute problem in the body. The most common culprit is a urinary tract infection. We'll discuss this subject more in chapter 4.

Increased confusion due to infections or other acute illnesses is called delirium. It's important for physicians to recognize delirium rather than assume confusion is due to the patient's dementia. An accurate diagnosis will hinge on your input about your loved one's baseline before the acute illness.

The most common medications given in AD are to slow memory loss. Donepezil (Aricept) and memantine (Namenda) have been shown to delay decline on average; that is, in large groups, those taking these drugs declined more slowly than those not taking them. This average result does not predict individual responses to these medications.

WHAT TO SAY

- "Look, Dad! It's our old neighbor, Bill." Look for ways to work in names and relationships without highlighting their memory loss.

- "It's dark now. Let's stay here tonight and go home in the morning." When they say they want to go home, they're often thinking of their childhood home. Telling them they are home doesn't help.

- "Grandma's at Aunt Virginia's house. She'll be home later." When they ask for dead loved ones, do *not* keep telling them that person passed away.

WHAT TO DO

- Avoid asking, "Do you remember … ?" This question puts your loved one on the spot. No one likes to feel dumb.

- Recognize that you can't pull someone out of their confusion by explaining to or arguing with them. If it's true in their mind, then it's true.

- Enter their world by going along with what they believe. You are not lying; it's a physician-advocated treatment to decrease their distress.

- If you notice an increase in their confusion over a few days, call your doctor to ask about urine testing. It could be a urinary tract infection.

- Know that changes in their routine and where they are will increase their confusion. Plan for this reaction when disruptions can't be avoided.

- Confusion increases anxiety. Reassure them that you're there and that they're safe.

WHAT TO ASK YOUR DOCTOR

- Could this confusion be from a urinary tract or other infection?

- Do you think this increased memory loss or confusion is caused by their dementia, or could it be a sign of delirium?

- See the "Questions to Ask About All Medications" sidebar (page 38) for additional questions.

Repetitive Actions

Few behaviors can pluck at a caregiver's nerves more than repetitive actions. When you've answered the same question eight times in the past half hour, it's hard to hear it again. Knowing that your loved one can't help it doesn't always make it easier.

Observing repetitive actions is another occasion to put on your detective hat. The goal is to guess what feelings may be behind the action. Anxiety, loneliness, and boredom are common triggers.

People with dementia may worry about what they're supposed to be doing. Or they may be hungry, thirsty, in pain, or in need of a bathroom visit. When language fails, repetitive behaviors may be the only signal you get.

Constantly following you around often means your loved one needs to see you to know you're there. Drumming fingers or pacing can signal boredom or excess energy. A stressful environment or overstimulation can cause repetitive behaviors.

Memory loss also comes into play here. Your loved one may not remember that they've already asked a question or that they just finished eating so it's not time to fix another meal.

It's easy to tell you to just be patient. This reaction usually comes from someone who's not in the line of fire. You may be able to decrease repetitive behaviors, but eliminating them is hard. This situation is a prime example of why caregivers must have time away on a regular basis.

WHAT TO SAY

- "Let's go for a walk." Repetitive actions can be the result of pent-up energy. Give them an outlet for it. The more active they are, the calmer they are likely to be.

- "I'm right here. I won't leave you." You may feel like a broken record by reassuring them over and over again. But with memory problems, they can't remember that you just told them they're safe. They need to hear it often.

- "Let's get you into the bathroom." All behavior has meaning. Pacing or other repetitive actions can be signaling an unmet need. When they start getting antsy, it is often a sign that they need to go to the bathroom but can't tell you with words.

- Use visual cues as reminders: big calendars, whiteboards, and clocks. Digital clocks that show the time, date, and part of the day (morning, afternoon, evening, night) are great.

- When memory fails, write notes and make signs. You can download a picture of just about anything to print out.

- When leaving your loved one with another caregiver, write down who is with them and when you'll be back.

- Wait until the day of an appointment or event to tell your loved one about it. They won't remember if you tell them in advance.

- Avoid telling them that they just asked you the same question, just had a snack, or just watered the plants. It will only increase their anxiety and the repetitive behavior.

- Provide plenty of reassurance and comfort, both in words and in touch.

- Try distracting them with a snack or activity. Give them something to do with their hands, like folding laundry, sorting a big jar of buttons by color, or holding a fidget blanket.

- Keep them physically active as much as you can. Moving to music always counts.

- Plan for regular breaks away from caregiving to ease your stress; a few hours twice a week is a good place to start. Expand from there. We'll talk more about this in chapter 9.

- Could these behaviors signal another problem beyond dementia?

- If so, what steps should I take?

- See the "Questions to Ask About All Medications" sidebar (page 38) for additional questions.

Sundowning

Sundowning is an experience of increased confusion and agitation late in the day. It starts in late afternoon and can last well into the night. Anxiety and aggression can develop. Some people hallucinate, seeing or hearing things that aren't really there.

There are multiple theories on what causes sundowning. A combination of factors makes the most sense. Dimming light and more shadows cause anxiety. They can also cause paranoia.

Fatigue is often a factor, in both the person with dementia and the caregiver. By late in the day, both of you may have exhausted your energy stores. Fatigue shows in our face, tone of voice, and posture. Your loved one's anxiety and confusion may increase in response to your fatigue.

The brain regulates sleep-wake cycles. When the brain fails, a person's internal clock can go haywire. They may have trouble knowing whether it's night or day. Medications can also affect the sleep-wake cycle.

A light sleeper with dementia may wake and believe their dream was reality. They may continue to act out their dream, which can lead to wandering or trying to leave the house. (See more on wandering on page 55.)

Sundowning can trigger placement in a care facility if left unchecked. Long-term sleep deprivation is used to torture prisoners of war. It effectively lowers the person's resistance to pressure. This result is no surprise to caregivers who can't remember the last time they got a full night's sleep.

- "Look, it's dark outside. It's time to be sleeping." Help them use long-instilled ideas to get their bearings. Darkness signals nighttime; snow signals cold; a set table signals time to eat.

- "This TV show is scaring me. Let's listen to some music." People with dementia will grasp only a fraction of what they see on TV and mix it up in their mind as real. To prevent your loved one from getting hyped up in the evening, screen what they're watching and hearing to protect them from things that can unnerve them when taken as real.

- "You've had a busy day. You must be tired." This statement is a clue that bedtime is approaching. Everyone likes to feel like they've accomplished something each day. Dementia doesn't erase that need. Positive reinforcement goes a long way. Emphasizing that they must be tired segues into bedtime.

- Keep the house well lit in the evening to minimize shadows and dark corners.

- Avoid a heavy meal in the evening. It is better to have a hearty meal at midday and a snack or light meal at dinnertime.

- Limit fluids after dinner to minimize bathroom trips in the night.

- Keep a routine schedule for waking and bedtime.

- Wear your loved one out during the day. Physical activity is your friend—the more, the merrier—and helps them sleep.

- Plan challenging tasks or trips at your loved one's best time of day, usually mornings.

- Limit the length of afternoon naps—unless you're the one napping, of course.

- Know that changes to and from daylight savings time can cause sundowning flare-ups.

- Plan ways to keep your home safe at night. You can use nightlights, locks, and motion sensors.

WHAT TO ASK YOUR DOCTOR

- What is the most likely reason for my loved one's changes late in the day?

- Could these changes come from an infection or other physical problem?

- Are there lighting changes I should make in the home that could help?

- See the "Questions to Ask About All Medications" sidebar (page 38) for additional questions.

Wandering

Wandering or getting lost is common in people with dementia. In AD, getting lost in a familiar place can be one of the first signs of illness. There are lots of reasons someone might wander.

It helps to look for reasons your loved one might be wandering. Stress and confusion in an unfamiliar place is one. Others are boredom; basic needs, like looking for the bathroom; or searching for someone or somewhere, such as home.

Here's something to remember: When people with dementia want to go "home," it's often their childhood home they are thinking of.

Wandering can result from following old routines. If Mom met the school bus at the corner every day for 15 years, she may head out now. Dad may be looking for the hardware store so he can fix those loose shingles. Never mind that it's 4:00 a.m.

Maintaining the safety of the wanderer is the top priority Losing track of a loved one is every caregiver's worst nightmare. Given that two-thirds of those with dementia will wander, it's right to be concerned. The potential for a crisis is always there.

Someone with dementia may not realize they're lost. They may not ask anyone for help. Or they may not remember their address or even their name. Most communities now have Safe Return programs operated through law enforcement or the Alzheimer's Association.

WHAT TO SAY

- "I would love to come along with you." When your loved one is determined to go, it can be impossible to redirect them. It's better to let them go. If they don't want you to come, walk a distance behind to make sure they're safe.

- "We have a bed here for tonight. I'm here with you. We'll go home in the morning. See, it's dark outside!" This is what is called a *fiblet,* or therapeutic fibbing. When someone is anxious and wants to go "home," you'll only make them more anxious by arguing that they're already home. You'll never win that argument. The kinder approach for both of you is to acknowledge their feelings and offer a plausible plan.

- "What's the first thing you'll do when you get home?" The desire to be in the childhood home reflects a feeling or comfort they long to return to. Talking about that home and what they love about it takes them there for a time. Follow this exchange with more questions to lead them into reminiscing.

- "Let's get you to the bathroom before I tuck you in." Consistent routines should mark important shifts in the day. Morning, bedtime, and mealtime routines provide structure for them to hold on to. Routines are clues to them about what comes next.

WHAT TO DO

- Look for clues about why your loved one might be wandering. All behavior has meaning. Wandering often signals an unmet need they can't communicate. Are they bored? Are they hungry? Are they lonely and missing "home"?

- Observe if wandering often happens around the same time of day.

- Plan reassuring activities around that time of day that will help them play out their memories. Walk Mom to the corner bus stop. Then remember it's a school holiday and come home.

- Distract and redirect with other tasks or activities your loved one enjoys.

- Order ID jewelry for your loved one and make sure they wear it. For some, this effort will be a losing battle. Just do what you can.

- Research personal location devices and apps, such as those listed in the Resources section at the back of this book (page 160). I like the work being done at Trackpatch.com. For those who won't wear a pendant or bracelet, this company offers a tea bag–size patch you put on the person's back just like a medication patch. It alerts you any time they go beyond set boundaries.

- Keep car keys, coats, and hats out of sight. If necessary, disable a vehicle or "take it in for repairs."

- Ask friends, family, and neighbors to call you if they see your loved one out alone.

- Modify your home to deter wandering.

- Write out an action plan in advance for if your loved one does get away from you.

  - List phone numbers of people who can help search.

  - Know if your loved one is right- or left-handed. People tend to turn in the direction of their dominant hand.

  - Keep a recent close-up photo and list of medical conditions to give police.

  - List places your loved one might seek out, like past homes or previous work addresses.

  - Contact the local Alzheimer's Association to ask about its Safe Return program for people with any type of dementia.

- If 15 minutes pass and you haven't found your loved one, call 911.

- What advice can you give me about keeping my loved one safe at home?

- What is your opinion on my loved one driving?

- What is the process to notify the Department of Motor Vehicles that you don't believe they are safe to drive?

- Are there other activities you would advise against for safety's sake?

- Do you feel medications might be necessary to prevent their wandering? (See the "Questions to Ask About All Medications" sidebar on page 38 for additional medication questions.)

How Are You Doing?

We've covered a lot of ground in this chapter. A loved one's mood changes and behaviors that are hard to understand are rough on any caregiver.

Considering all of the symptoms we might one day face is overwhelming. Or should I say *paralyzing*? Caring for a loved one with dementia is like running a long-distance race. We have to do it one step at a time.

Feelings of guilt plague most caregivers. You want to do your very best for your loved one. You want them to have the best care and the highest quality of life possible.

But no one was born knowing how to be an expert. I promise that you will make mistakes and choose what will later prove to be the wrong paths. But you'll survive, and your loved one will still love you deep in their heart of hearts.

Chances are you haven't seen a family caring for someone with dementia. The prevalence of dementia is a relatively new phenomenon. So, what do you do without role models?

You do exactly what you're doing right now. You educate yourself. The more you know, the more confidence you can have. Seek out reading materials that bolster your spirits. There are books with daily inspirations for everyone. Find one that speaks to you.

Keep in mind that surviving this role means being good to yourself. Seek out encouragement from those who love you. The path you've chosen to follow is extraordinarily challenging. Go easy on yourself.

Here's a routine you can try this week. Write down the five senses: sight, hearing, taste, smell, and touch. For each sense, name two things you love. You now have a list of 10 delights. At the end of each day, look at your list. How many delights did you give yourself that day? Make a goal of not letting a day pass without indulging a minimum of two senses with something you love.

CHAPTER FOUR

COMMON DAILY LIVING CHANGES

CARL

"I already took a shower today." "I told you, Carl. You haven't taken a shower all week. You're starting to smell. Why do you have to make this so hard? It's ridiculous." Judy threw up her hands in disgust and headed for the backyard.

Carl wondered why his wife wanted him to take two showers in the same day. He didn't like it when she got angry. Just then, he heard music come on the TV and went to see what it was.

Judy's hands were shaking so much that she could barely light her cigarette. She'd quit smoking six months ago, but today was too overwhelming to handle. She didn't know if she was angrier with Carl or herself.

It had started that morning. Judy came down to the kitchen to find Carl pouring milk over a bowl of leftover green beans. He then proceeded to eat them with his fingers. She supposed she should be glad he was eating anything. Carl stood 6 feet 2 inches and was down to 170 pounds.

That afternoon, their daughter, Jenny, called to say something came up and she wasn't going to be able to sit with her dad on Saturday. Judy's plans for a break went out the window. "Good thing I never have anything come up," she said under her breath.

When Judy got off the phone, she walked into the living room. There sat Carl, grinning at The Price Is Right. He was oblivious to the puddle of urine under his chair. That's when the fight over taking a shower had started.

Judy knew Carl couldn't help how he was. Every day, she told herself she wasn't going to lose her temper today. She was going to remember all those things she read online. She was going to get it right. "Oh, hell," she thought. "I guess today isn't that day." She put out her cigarette and dragged herself back inside. It was time to make dinner.

Eating and Nutrition

Good nutrition for those with dementia can be a hot-button topic. Our bodies respond to a well-balanced diet with more energy and physical ease. The same is true for people who develop dementia. But when, if ever, does it become pointless to restrict the diet of one with a terminal condition?

Most people with dementia experience a decrease in appetite, often from a decline in sensory perception. Smell, flavor, and presentation contribute to desiring food. Brain disease and normal aging dull these senses. The ability to distinguish flavors fades, with sweetness being the last flavor to go.

Memory loss and time confusion don't help, either. Your loved one may not remember to eat or may forget that they just had a large meal. Frustration with how to use a fork or not recognizing foods creates anxiety. A person may be hungry but refuse to eat because they don't remember how to use utensils.

Then there's the person whose brain no longer signals when to stop eating. This person is constantly looking for something to nibble on. They can no more help that urge than they can help forgetting what day it is. It's a symptom of brain failure. You may need to lock the pantry or refrigerator. Be sure to keep snacks easily accessible, putting out only what your loved one needs.

Adequate fluid intake is a challenge for many of us, but for a person with dementia, fluids are critical. Fluids help flush out the urinary tract, which decreases infections; they help maintain adequate blood pressure to prevent falls; and they promote digestion and reduce constipation.

Preventing dehydration in someone with dementia is a daily challenge. They forget there's a glass of water right next to them. They don't always experience thirst. Beverages that used to satisfy now have no flavor. Constant nagging to drink is frustrating for both the one with dementia and the one nagging. It's enough to drive a caregiver a little bit crazy.

People with dementia will eventually lose their ability to swallow. Eating and drinking require signals from the brain to activate strong muscles in the neck and throat. When those signals fail, knowing what to do with food or fluids in their mouth also fails.

At this stage, a well-intentioned but uninformed physician may offer a feeding tube. The American Geriatrics Society issued a position statement in 2014 against using feeding tubes in advanced dementia. Multiple studies prove that feeding tubes do not extend life expectancy. They only cause more suffering in the time that is left.

WHAT TO SAY

- "Look, Dad. It's pot roast and mashed potatoes tonight, your favorites!" Announce what is on the plate you set before your loved one.

- "Grandma, would you like lemonade or juice?" Give your loved one two choices for food or drink. Asking "What would you like for dinner?" involves too many options. Narrow it down for them.

- "Mom, take a few sips of your tea. The doctor said it's very important to keep you healthy." Cue them at least once an hour to take a few sips of a drink.

- Make mealtime a calm and unhurried time. Turn off the TV and any other noise sources. Soft music can decrease anxiety and promote better intake. Keep the tabletop clear during meals to prevent distraction. Eat with your loved one to model how it's done.

- Serve no more than three foods at a time on the plate. Serve small portions, with the option for seconds. Try to vary colors and textures in a meal. Cut food into bite-size pieces in advance. Doing so promotes dignity, versus cutting it up for them at the table.

- Use red plates. Studies show that using a red plate can increase food intake. Try with red plastic plates before buying new dinnerware.

- When eating out, consider these tips:

  o Try to schedule the meal outside of peak busy hours for restaurants.

  o Ask to be seated in the quietest area to minimize distractions.

  o Pick two items from the menu to offer to your loved one. Look for finger foods if using utensils is an issue.

  o Consider ordering from the kids' menu for serving sizes that won't overwhelm. Or you can ask for portions to be divided between a plate and a to-go box before being served.

  o Carry small cards you can discreetly slip to the server. They may read, "My companion is living with dementia. They may react slowly or seem confused. Your patience and understanding will help greatly."

You can print these cards yourself or order them online from any printing service. Carry them wherever you go to alert others to the situation. They've greased a lot of wheels for me.

- Use insulated cups with lids to prevent spills. Use bowls, which are easier to eat from than plates. Spoons are easier than forks. Switch to finger foods when utensils become too confusing. Do an online search for "finger foods" to get ideas.

- Offer their favorites every day if that's what they want. If they refuse any foods other than sweets, remember that eating sweets is better than eating nothing. Sweet is a taste they still can enjoy. Ice cream is your friend. Mix it with a little protein powder and full-fat milk for milkshakes that count.

WHAT TO ASK YOUR DOCTOR

- Are there any vitamins or other supplements that I should be giving my loved one?

- Are smoothies or meal replacement shakes safe for them?

- My loved one has diabetes. Should I keep them from eating sweets? What if sweets are all they will eat?

- Would speech therapy help their swallowing problems?

Incontinence

Incontinence is a symptom of brain failure that most caregivers dread. For some families, this symptom is the tipping point for seeking full-time facility care. Incontinence evokes difficult emotions in both our loved ones and us. They often feel humiliated, and we feel embarrassed for them.

Incontinence usually develops gradually. Sudden, full incontinence may be due to a different medical problem, which you should speak with a doctor about. Urinary incontinence tends to come first, with bowel incontinence delayed by months or even years.

In some cases, you can delay incontinence with toilet training. Escort your loved one to the toilet every two hours during waking hours. Encourage them to sit on the commode even if they feel like they don't need to go. Turning on running water may help induce urination. Try the universal battle cry if you meet resistance: "The doctor says it's important for you to do this."

WHAT TO SAY

- "I know this is hard for you; I'm just glad you will let me help you." Sometimes a simple statement is all you can say when your loved one is embarrassed.

- "At least you're not constipated." A joke can highlight the silver lining and lighten the mood.

- "Let's go for a walk when we're done." Taking the focus off their embarrassment may lead to more comfortable conversation.

WHAT TO DO

- If your loved one goes from being continent to complete incontinence in a few days, have their physician evaluate them. Incontinence due to dementia rarely develops suddenly.

- If your loved one resists wearing incontinence briefs (please don't call them diapers), you may need to remove their underwear from their dresser. Fill that space with disposable briefs.

- Buy only a small supply of briefs at first. Try a few brands before finding one that fits and gets the job done.

- Consider buying briefs and wipes online once you know which brand you want. Shopping online can save money and provides the convenience of home delivery.

- If your loved one has Medicaid coverage, check with their eligibility worker to see if incontinence products are covered. In some states, they are.

- Add 1 cup of white vinegar plus 1 cup of baking soda to your detergent to cut stubborn odors in clothing. It works as well as more costly cleaning products.

- Gather supplies you may eventually need. Gloves and face masks are in the pharmacy aisle. I know it sounds awful, but you may thank me later. A small jar of menthol ointment can help. A dab just below your nose can mask difficult odors.

- Keep an emergency kit in the car for accidents away from home. Include a complete change of clothes: top and bottom plus footwear. You also want two plastic bags, one for soiled clothing and one for disposable items. Don't forget gloves and wipes.

- Do whatever you have to do to avoid scolding a loved one for something they can't prevent. Even in advanced dementia, incontinence remains a source of embarrassment for many.

- Do the best you can to wash your loved one's hands after an incontinent episode. Keep a nail brush by the sink. If they have "painted" any surfaces, it's because they didn't know what was on their hands. They tried to wipe it off as best as they knew how. Keep fingernails short to promote cleanliness.

- Keep hand sanitizer around the house and in your purse or car. Keep a bottle anywhere eating happens. Rubbing their hands with sanitizer is often easier than getting them to use soap and water.

WHAT TO ASK YOUR DOCTOR

- Could the incontinence be from something besides dementia?

- Are there any medications that might cause incontinence? (See the "Questions to Ask About All Medications" sidebar on page 38 for additional medication questions.)

- How often should my loved one have a bowel movement?

- What can I do to prevent constipation?

- What should I do if they develop constipation?

Giving Medication

Getting someone with dementia to take medications can be a challenge. They aren't trying to be difficult; it's just something unpleasant for them. They know that no amount of pudding can block the nasty taste of medicine. They don't understand why they need to take medication. And it may be hard to swallow pills.

Many medications now come in liquid form or as a cream or patch to absorb through the skin. Don't assume all is lost if you can't get something into your loved one. Check with their doctor or pharmacist for alternatives.

One important habit to break is explaining things in detail to your loved one. We must wrap our minds around how easily extra words confuse them, especially when it comes to medications.

When your loved one balks at taking medicine, the more you talk, the more likely they are to dig in their heels because they can't understand what you are saying. The more confused they feel, the more resistant they'll be.

It's hard to get someone who's already agitated to take something to calm down. When emotions are running high, yours and theirs, taking a pill may be the last thing your loved one will do. It's better to watch for signs of trouble approaching and try to give the pill before things escalate.

WHAT TO SAY

- "It's chocolate time!" That's right: Bribe them with the promise of a treat afterward. You're creating positive reinforcement. If you're consistent with this tactic, they'll eventually associate the pills with the treat and be less resistant.

- "It's time to take our medicine." Try the buddy system. If you take medications, do it together. If you don't, fake it with a small candy or mint.

- *Nothing.* Yes, I mean say nothing. Bob DeMarco of the Alzheimer's Reading Room described giving his mother medications. He'd bring out the ice cream. Then he'd hold one pill at a time out to her. And he'd hand her a lightweight glass of water once she put the pill in her mouth. He remained silent no matter what until the last pill was gone. Then it was time to celebrate. "Great job, Mom! Let's have some ice cream."

- Consult a pharmacist or your physician before crushing any pills to be sure it's safe to do so.

- Pick up a pill cutter or crusher at any pharmacy. Some pharmacies will cut pills in half for you to match a doctor's order. It doesn't hurt to ask.

- Use a pillbox, even if your loved one takes only one pill a day. A pillbox eliminates wondering later on if you gave today's dose.

- When giving medications, your mantra should be "Talk less; gesture more."

- Pick your battles. Start with giving the pills that matter most. Medicines for difficult symptoms should be a priority. If your loved one decides they've had enough halfway through, you can try the rest of the pills later.

- Pudding, applesauce, or softened ice cream can help with swallowing. Be sure to put the medicine in only a spoonful. The less they have to eat to get the pill, the better.

- Mix crushed pills with jam, not jelly. Jam has small bits of fruit, so small crumbs of a pill blend in.

- Check your nonverbal messages. If your frustration comes out in the tone or volume of your voice, it will make things worse.

- If you aren't getting anywhere, let someone else in the household try. The sweet grandchild may succeed when you don't. It's nothing personal.

- If you or your loved one is stuck or exasperated, leave it. You can try again in 10 or 15 minutes. A battle of the wills is not what you want them to associate with taking their medicine.

- What can I try to get them to take their medications?
- Could you go over their medicines with me to show which ones are most important?
- Could you tell me the purpose of each medication and whether we can eliminate it?
- Are there any medications my loved one has been on longer than is usually recommended? (A reasonable doctor will welcome your interest. If they balk at this question, it's their ego and not you that is out of line.)
- Are any of these medicines unsafe to break or crush before giving them?
- Are any of these medicines available as a liquid or in a patch or cream?
- My loved one has been on Alzheimer's medicines for over a year. Is it recommended to keep taking them? (No studies exist that show these medicines help for longer than one year.)

Mobility

Dementia affects gait, balance, and muscle strength, resulting in a decrease in mobility. Walking is a complex function in which the brain sends impulses or commands to the muscles to move. Brain failure affects the brain's perception of the environment and impairs the commands it sends to muscles.

Gait refers to how someone walks. It includes how the feet move and how weight is shifted from one leg to another.

Dementia may cause someone to shuffle their feet across the floor or to have trouble initiating each step. Telling someone to just lift their feet is often beyond what their brain can process.

Balance is our ability to maintain our body weight in an upright position. It requires an awareness of the environment and of our body parts. This awareness originates in the brain. Responding to changes in the environment starts in the brain. As brain disease progresses, it's more difficult to stay balanced.

Muscle strength is affected by dementia indirectly. Changes in vision and balance combined with a fear of falling can lead to less walking. The use-it-or-lose-it principle says that less walking means decreased muscle strength.

Mobility can also decline due to medications and their side effects. Many medications cause dizziness, making it hard to maintain balance. Others can cause drops in blood pressure upon standing, which may cause an instance of blacking out or seeing stars with a loss of balance and a fall.

Daily physical activity is key to delaying mobility issues for as long as possible. Physical therapy, especially in the early stages of dementia, can help. Occupational therapists can advise how to adapt the environment and suggest walking patterns to promote mobility.

WHAT TO SAY

- "We haven't been for a walk today. Let's see how it feels outside." You can provide positive reinforcement with a calendar. At the end of a walk or other physical activity, make an X for that date. See how many Xs in a row you can mark.

- "It's too cold to go outside today. Let's try these exercises the physical therapist showed us." Physical and occupational therapists are primarily there to train people and to set up a program you can use well into the future.

- "I remember this song. I bet I can outdance you on this one." Dancing is movement to music. It doesn't have to be coordinated or syncopated to work.

- "Look. I found some exercises we can do sitting down." You'll find a friend in online videos. Search online for "chair exercises" to find a variety of videos to follow.

- "Pull on that bar, Mom. Feel how secure it is." Fear of falling will require your encouragement and cuing for them to know that they are safe.

WHAT TO DO

- Walk through your home looking for potential barriers to free movement.

- Learn and follow the exercises any therapists provide to promote stability and muscle strength.

- If your loved one uses a cane for balance, put up hooks in places they often sit. This keeps the cane off the floor where it's a major trip hazard.

- If your loved one uses a walker, decorate it. Decorations make it easier to see than bland gray metal. Ribbons, artificial flowers, a walker bag, or a basket should all be securely fastened to prevent becoming a hazard. Nursing homes that have implemented decorations saw an increase in the use of walkers and many fewer falls.

- If your loved one gets tired or winded as they move with a walker, get one with a seat they can rest on. Make sure it has easy-to-use brakes. These brakes *must* be engaged when getting on and off.

- Never push someone who's sitting on one of these walkers. It takes almost nothing for them to tip over, throwing the passenger on the ground. It's extremely dangerous, even for just a few feet.

- What kinds of physical activity do you think would be most helpful to my loved one?

- Would physical therapy and occupational therapy benefit my loved one right now?

- Do any of the medications my loved one is taking increase their risk for falls?

- Should I be concerned about their blood pressure dropping when they stand up? What can I do to minimize the chance of that happening?

Personal Hygiene

Personal hygiene is a major challenge for someone with dementia. People who always cared about their appearance eventually lose all interest. Their awareness of body odor or soiled clothing disappears over time. It can be shocking to see what our loved ones will accept or are unaware of.

We were all taught at an early age that the bathroom is a place to discreetly take care of our hygiene needs. Needing help in this area is a blow to anyone's sense of independence. Embarrassment and frustration can run high for both our loved ones and us. Fortunately, there are ways to get the job done without all the rancor.

Most people with dementia resist bathing with unparalleled determination. Physical and emotional discomfort are at the root of their resistance. Success means guessing what the causes of discomfort might be and acting to minimize them.

Pain in arthritic joints can flare with standing or lifting legs in and out of a tub. When the brain is on the blink, normal room and water temperatures may feel uncomfortable. Fear of falling is common. Shower water hitting the skin can sting. Washing hair means water near the face and can feel like drowning.

Toileting, brushing their teeth, washing their face, or getting dressed are all hurdles for people with dementia. Each of these tasks includes many individual steps. Remembering the steps and the order to take them can easily be beyond our loved one's abilities.

WHAT TO SAY

- "Here's your washcloth. Let's wipe your face." Encourage them to do as much as they can. Use short instructions and allow time for them to process each step before giving them the next step.

- "You have a doctor's appointment this afternoon. I know you want to clean up for that." It's okay to stretch the truth (therapeutic fibbing) on any occasion that helps get them into the shower. If your loved one later asks about the outing or visitors, reply that it had to be rescheduled.

- "It's time for your spa treatment." Putting a positive spin on bathing can help. Set up the bathroom to fit the occasion. Soft music, candles, or soaps with fragrances they like may help.

- "You did it for me, Mom. Now it's my turn to do it for you." Reassuring them that you're willing to take on embarrassing tasks matters.

- "Let's have ice cream when we finish here." Anticipating a reward can disrupt their focus on a difficult job in the bathroom.

- Keep hygiene tasks as close as you can to your loved one's former habits. If they preferred a bath over a shower, stick with that. Were they a morning or an evening bather? Did they get manicures or pedicures at a salon?

- Daily wash-ups at the sink and two showers a week are enough for most people. Hit the most important areas first in case they balk midway. Face, armpits, under large breasts, genitals, and rear need daily attention with a sink bath. The rest can wait.

- Pay attention to their nails. Keep fingernails short. Keep a nail brush handy in any bathroom they use. Visit a salon or a podiatrist to keep toenails in check. If you're going DIY on toenails, soak their feet in warm water first to make clipping easier.

- Keep sanitizer anywhere that food is eaten. Make it a new tradition that everyone has to have a few drops to clean their hands before eating.

- Prepare the bathroom before escorting your loved one in for bathing. Make sure the room is warmed up first. Have all supplies, like soap and towels, lined up in reach of the tub or shower. Have clothing and briefs on hand to dress in the bathroom, where it is warm.

- Using a colored tub mat or nonslip strips in the bottom of the tub decreases fear from being unable to see the bottom, a common problem as vision changes.

- You can play up the notion of a spa treatment, avoiding the dreaded "B word" (*bath*, not the other one). Light a few candles, diffuse lavender oil, and play soft music.

- Modesty can be maintained during bathing. Let them wear underwear into the shower to limit their exposure. You can pull the underwear to the side to wash that area. Some caregivers wear a bathing suit when giving a bath, which allows standing close, easing your loved one's fear of falling.

- Have enough towels in the house to supply the U.S. Army. Use several towels after bathing: one around their shoulders, one across their chest, one across their lap, and one for their hair. If they have dry or fragile skin, try to dab gently rather than rub dry.

- Throw towels into the dryer for a few minutes before using. Few things feel better than warm towels after bathing.

- Using body lotion daily on most of their skin will help prevent skin tears and pressure wounds. Moisturizers with shea butter work best.

- Keep skin clean and dry as much as possible. Any area that is warm, dark, and damp is going to grow fungus. Urine and feces have enzymes that damage the skin. It's impossible to keep an incontinent person dry all the time; just do the best you can.

- My go-to cream to protect skin is cheap and effective. Pick up store-brand hydrocortisone cream plus athlete's foot cream (anything with clotrimazole listed as a primary ingredient). Mix equal parts of the creams together on your fingertips. Apply a thin layer anywhere you want to protect their skin. A thick layer only wastes cream without added benefit. You can use this cream with each brief change and after bathing. It works well under large breasts.

- Consider hiring a home health aide to come in twice a week to shower, shave, buff, and fluff your loved one. It's a good way to start introducing other caregivers. A male caregiver may have better luck with men. People will often do things for someone they see as a professional that they won't do for us. It's worth a shot.

WHAT TO ASK YOUR DOCTOR

- Is there any equipment you would recommend to use at home for hygiene?

- Would an evaluation by a home occupational therapist be possible? (Occupational therapists specialize in techniques to accommodate decreased abilities.)

- Are there any special precautions we should take with my loved one's skin? How can we prevent pressure sores?

Safety at Home

It's natural to think of baby- or puppy-proofing a home. When dementia comes calling, we need to take many of the same precautions. It seems like hazards are at every turn.

Falls are one of the first things that come to mind when we consider home safety. We also must guard against wandering. And more than one person with dementia has started a fire by leaving pans on the stove or popcorn in the microwave for too long.

Brain failure affects people's vision, depth perception, balance, and safety judgment. It tells them the bottle of aspirin is candy. It gives them delusions about where they are and where they ought to be. It's up to us to protect them the best we know how.

With all the ways dementia changes our loved ones, it's hard to think of all the possible hazards on our own. Luckily, there are lots of checklists out there to download and print. I've included one in the Resources section at the back of this book (page 160). Some home health companies, insurance agents, and local fire departments provide in-home safety assessments.

Clutter is often an issue for the elderly. Half a century in the same house can mean 50 years of accumulated furniture, containers, clothes—the list goes on and on. In excess, these items can quickly become a source of falls, fires, and disease.

The challenge is balancing the need for safety with the emotional needs of our loved ones. Dementia highlights how fragile their ties to the past may be. Their need to feel independent often means resisting intervention. "No child of mine is going to tell me what I can have in my own home." Sound familiar?

While we are talking about safety, let me mention driving. Talk with the physician about whether your loved one should be driving. They should be able to advise you on ways to enforce a change. Every state has its own laws for reporting someone who shouldn't be driving. Most won't reveal the source of the report if certain guidelines are followed.

Taking away the car keys is a heartbreaking milestone but one that may save lives. Dementia care programs at some major medical centers offer driver testing and rehabilitation. Conduct a search online for "driver rehabilitation" in your area. Or contact the nearest teaching hospital to ask if they have a specialized memory care program.

Choosing your battles in dementia care is important. But battles over safety are hard to avoid. The truth is we will never eliminate all hazards for our loved one. Many times, we have to just do what we can and hope for the best.

WHAT TO SAY

- "Which coffee table is your favorite? What do you like about it?" Identifying items that your loved one likes most can help them let go of others.

- "I remember when you got these dishes. I'd love it if each of us had a place setting to remember them by." Scaling down allows holding onto a memory without needing entire collections. It honors the memory while removing one more clutter hazard.

- "Would you like your seat in the shower to have a back like a chair?" Including them in planning when they are able to respond reinforces feelings of independence.

WHAT TO DO

- Consult the Alzheimer's Association's home safety checklist. The website is listed in the Resources section (page 160). The checklist gives you room-by-room details of what you can do to eliminate hazards.

- Have a professional install modifications, like grab bars. The last thing you want is for something to come off in your loved one's hand.

- Consult a locksmith for options to prevent your loved one from leaving without making doors difficult for you to use.

- You may find used equipment at some medical equipment stores or websites. Try the equipment yourself before purchasing to make sure there are no mechanical issues.

- Consider having a home physical therapist or occupational therapist go through the home to recommend changes for safety. Or call your local fire department to ask if it offers a similar service.

- Do an online search for "reporting an impaired driver" in your state. This search should direct you to the laws and procedures you need to follow to get an unsafe loved one off the road.

- If your loved one drives off and you're worried about hazardous driving, call 911. Be prepared to provide the vehicle description and plate number if you have it. Emphasize that the driver has dementia and may not understand all commands.

- Ask other families in support groups for safety ideas they implemented or ways to end a loved one's driving.

WHAT TO ASK YOUR DOCTOR

- Would it benefit my loved one to have a physical or occupational therapist see them at home for a safety assessment?

- Are there community resources you know of to help with home modifications for the disabled?

- Is my loved one safe to drive? Is there a way to inform the Department of Motor Vehicles of this change? How does the agency respond?

- Do you know of any driver rehabilitation programs for people with dementia?

Sex and Intimacy

All humans need loving, safe relationships as well as affectionate touch. This need is as true for someone with dementia as for anyone else. But dementia often changes a person's level of desire and sexual behaviors. If you're both caregiver and partner to someone living with dementia, you will face changes in your relationship. Suffering in silence won't help either of you.

Research shows that most home-dwelling people with dementia who have a spouse or partner are sexually active. Age, stage of brain failure, and which brain areas are diseased affect how intimacy is expressed. Emotional changes in both partners affect desire and behaviors as much as physical changes do.

In the early stages of dementia, changes are mostly due to emotional shifts in the relationship. Feelings of inadequacy, rejection, and guilt are common. *Will he still want me? What if it upsets her? How will I know if it's okay to start something? Is this behavior coming from the person I love or from something weird happening in their brain? Are changes I won't like waiting down the road?*

A drop in desire that bothers either partner warrants medical attention. The decrease may not be associated with dementia at all. Hormonal imbalances, depression, and many medications may be to blame. The only way to know is to be evaluated by a physician.

An acceleration of desire is a change that many partners fear. Increased desire and decreased inhibition do happen together. This change can lead to behaviors a person would not have exhibited in the past. Someone with desires may not remember how they've addressed these needs before.

As brain disease progresses, signals get crossed in response to sensations. What looks like sexual behavior may be due to needing to go to the bathroom, being bored, or feeling physically uncomfortable.

When a spouse or partner moves into a care facility, new challenges often occur. By that time, the dementia is well progressed. It can be easy to mistake another resident for one's own spouse. Normal needs for physical closeness minus normal inhibition may lead to making advances with the care staff. Public masturbation happens, often due to boredom more than any sexual desire.

When a person with dementia loses orientation to themselves and their situation, the question of consent arises. Can someone with advanced dementia consent to sex? It's a legal and ethical question that's hard to answer. Consumer, legal, medical, and academic groups are seeking to define consent in practical ways.

Dementia caregiving for a spouse or partner is vastly different from caring for a parent. The changes in physical and emotional closeness account for much of the difference. Acknowledging these unique challenges and looking to others for support are the healthiest response for both caregiver and care recipient.

WHAT TO SAY

- "I don't want to lose you." Talking about our fears with our loved one while they still understand is important. This statement opens the door for them to express their own concerns.

- "Can I have a cuddle?" Sex is not the only way to satisfy a need for physical closeness. Initiating contact in non-sexual ways can benefit you both.

- "You're hurting me." Your loved one with dementia won't always know how to express themselves. Their behavior has nothing to do with you; it's the result of brain failure. If you ever feel you are in danger, reach out to your doctor or call 911.

WHAT TO DO

- Look for ways to include physical touch in your daily routines. Holding hands, hugging, and massage can satisfy the need for contact.

- Keep up other habits that contribute to closeness with your loved one, like taking walks together, sharing a meal, or watching a movie together.

- Keep your loved one as physically active as possible to burn off some of their extra energy.

- Use distraction and redirection to shift focus from undesired behaviors.

- Try to remember that changes in your loved one are not personal. Talking with a friend or advisor about your feelings prevents you from keeping them bottled up.

- If your loved one is in a care facility and you develop concerns, talk with the nursing staff about ways to manage the situation.

- Educate yourself on sexuality and the problems you may encounter. Look for reliable sources online, such as university- or government-based websites, for tips and ideas.

WHAT TO ASK YOUR DOCTOR

- Is there a way to control my spouse's incessant demands for sex?

- If doing so means medication, is it safe for them to take it? (See the "Questions to Ask About All Medications" sidebar on page 38 for additional medication questions.)

- How should I deal with a situation if I am scared of what my loved one might do?

How Are You Doing?

Daily living with someone with dementia is probably unlike anything you've previously experienced. No two days are the same. Uncertainty at what may come next is enough to demoralize the strongest caregiver. If you're not feeling afraid and overwhelmed right now, you are either in denial or under the influence of too many adult beverages.

Don't let the dash of humor fool you. Accomplishing the care discussed in this chapter makes getting a Harvard law degree look easy. Your emotions are bound to be racing from one feeling to another and back again.

Keep in mind that feelings are not facts. On the days you feel like a failure, it doesn't mean you are a failure. Stay with the facts. The facts are that you haven't abandoned your loved one, you are doing a thousand times better than you feel you are, and there's always hope that tomorrow will be better.

You're under pressure that's hard for others to imagine or for you to describe. But you're not alone. There are millions of others out there right now trying to find their way, too. Connecting with some of them can be therapeutic and comforting.

You'll find groups online where caregivers can vent, ask for advice, laugh at themselves, or just read the trials of others. This self-care is available anywhere at any time you need a boost. And we all need a boost every day we call ourselves caregivers.

Whenever you need it, here's a simple exercise you can use to slow down anxious thoughts. Do your best to hide, or find a spot where you won't be interrupted for five minutes. Sit or lie down in a position that feels comfortable.

Close your eyes. Take three deep breaths in through your nose and out through your mouth. With each breath, breathe in calm; breathe out fear. Breathe in calm. Breathe out fear. Now, breathe normally to proceed.

Keep your eyes closed until you have heard five distinct sounds. If you live near a busy road, passing cars don't count. Listen for the ticking clock, the hum of the air conditioner, the muted sound of the television at the other end of the house, sounds you may not normally notice. I almost always find that I have to listen so carefully to hear five sounds that I forget all else for that moment. Moments of peace will save us over time, but we often have to create them for ourselves.

CHAPTER FIVE

FINANCIAL AND LEGAL DECISIONS

KUMIKO

"I think you're totally overreacting. Mom was great when I was there. I'm going to call her doctor. If Mom wants to stay in her apartment, I don't see why you want to drag her out of it." Kumiko took a deep breath and bit her tongue. Her brother, Hiroshi, had visited for a whole three days this year. Now he was an expert on how bad their mother's memory was and the best plan for her.

Kumiko got off the phone and poured herself a glass of wine. It was probably a good thing that her brother was three states away right now. If he were here, she might need bail money by morning. Hiroshi had always been the hot shot. Always sure he knew just what everyone around him should be doing. But he was wrong about Mom. Kumiko was sure of it.

She opened a desk drawer and pulled out a thick folder labeled "Legal." Her power-of-attorney papers sat on top of the pile. A sense of peace washed over Kumiko. She reread how she was the one to make her mother's care decisions. Looking at her mother's scrawled signature, she could feel her mother's love. Mom knew what Hiroshi was like. Her trip to the lawyer last spring had settled that Kumiko's judgment would not be overruled.

Finances

In the weeks after a dementia diagnosis, medical needs feel paramount. We have so many questions about the diagnosis, doctors, and medications. We're eager to learn as much as we can about the disease.

Although these issues are important, medicine's ability to affect your loved one's outcome is limited. Actions with the most benefit for the future are not medical; they're financial and legal. And the sooner you address these issues, the better off you and your loved one will be.

Talking about money at this time may seem callous to some. But financial matters have often already begun to slip. Overdue bills, bounced checks, and excessive spending may be the first symptoms of brain illness.

When money judgment falters, a person in early dementia is vulnerable. Scams targeting them abound. Sketchy offers to do outdoor work for cash in advance are common. Insomnia leads to watching late night TV with all its offers of life-changing products and easy ordering. Scammers may pose as a grandchild on the phone and ask for money to post bail. Others will threaten the listener with being arrested if an immediate payment over the phone isn't made.

Protecting your loved one can be a complicated task. Seizing their credit cards and checkbook ranks up there with taking the car keys. No one wants to lose their independence. We don't want to take it away, but the potential cost of inaction is much too high to avoid these discussions.

Planning for future care costs is another reality we're better off facing early on. Future costs will hinge on how much care your loved one needs and how long it's needed. Predicting those two factors is hard with dementia. But we can look at averages of what others with a similar diagnosis experienced. Educated guessing is better than groping in the dark.

You may think financial planners and setting up trusts are only for the affluent. Not so. The fewer resources available, the more important it is to plan carefully. Financial planners are just one source of help. Other resources are available at lower costs or for free.

Very few of us have unlimited resources for future care. Fears of financial ruin can tempt us to pull a Scarlett O'Hara: "I'll think about that tomorrow." Delaying only causes unnecessary suffering. The sooner we nail down a basic financial plan, the sooner we realize we have options.

WHAT TO SAY

- "Mom, I'll just take these and put them in order. Then I'll bring them back for you." Scoop up any mail you see. Then you can find out what accounts are open. Don't ask if you can take the mail if you aren't prepared to take no for an answer.

- "Good thing you're a veteran, Dad." The U.S. Department of Veterans Affairs has a program called Aid and Attendance that will pay up to a few thousand dollars a month toward care.

- "I'm so relieved we bought that long-term care policy when we did." Once a dementia diagnosis is on the books, purchasing long-term care insurance is not possible.

- "I'll just pay the bills for now until we get straight with the bank." Portraying help as a temporary measure can increase the chances that your loved one will accept your offer.

- Obtain a durable power of attorney. This authorization needs to be in place before you can make transactions on your loved one's behalf.

- Decrease the limit on credit cards to minimize over-spending. If the problem persists, cancel the cards.

- Talk with the bank manager of your loved one's accounts. Ask if there are alerts you can receive for low balances, large cash withdrawals, or purchases. Ask if the bank has its own required power-of-attorney form, as some banks will honor only a document that originates at the bank.

- Add your name to your loved one's accounts to avoid being blocked from them when your loved one dies. A power of attorney automatically ceases at the assigner's death. If there's not a co-owner on a bank account, it's frozen pending probate.

- Gather account numbers, balances, and values for any property, cash, retirement accounts, stocks and bonds, other assets, and all debts.

- Clarify what health, long-term care, and life insurance policies are active. If a policy was recently canceled for nonpayment, contact the carrier to see if you can back-pay premiums to reinstate it. It's a long shot but not totally unheard of.

- Write down the sources and amounts of monthly income for all household members. Keep a copy in your care binder that you created earlier for keeping medical his-tory and documents.

- List routine expenses, including both monthly and inter-mittent expenses. Keep a copy in your binder.

- Search online to find resources with reliable information on daily, monthly, and annual costs of long-term care in your area. Check the Resources section (page 160) for helpful websites to get started.

- Make an appointment with a financial advisor. Ask friends for recommendations. For middle- and low-income families, visit the Association for Financial Counseling and Planning Education online. This nonprofit focuses on financial education and planning, not on selling financial products. Find it at AFCPE.org.

- If you can't or prefer not to use a professional advisor, contact local agencies that may offer help planning for costs of dementia care. Many chapters of the Alzheimer's Association offer help. Do an online search for "area board for aging" for your area. Some boards provide insurance counseling for elders that could help you. The local department of social services and Social Security Administration offices can help determine benefits your loved one may be entitled to.

- Talk with a certified public accountant or financial planner about the tax implications of serious chronic illness. You'll want to know about deductions allowed. Many states have tax breaks for caregivers.

- If you don't have access to finance professionals, find your state AARP chapter via the national website. AARP offers free tax counseling and tax preparation for elders. Membership is not required.

- Educate yourself on Medicaid rules for your state. Rules are complex and may require action long before you expect to apply. Search online for "Medicaid requirements" in your state. Stick with sites that end in .gov or .org to get the most accurate information. Medicaid.gov is the federal website, and it also has a lot of information you'll find helpful.

- Consult the National Council on Aging's website Benefitscheckup.org to find federal, state, and local programs your loved one may qualify for. This site keeps a huge database of programs and their requirements sorted by location.

- Would a revocable trust help preserve my loved one's assets?

- What financial steps should I take now? In six months? In a year?

- If I have to leave my job to care for my loved one, can I charge my loved one for my care? How can I protect my own financial future?

- If my spouse needs Medicaid to pay for their care, what would happen to our home? To our car? Are there federal laws to help a spouse hang on to these assets?

- If I move in with my parent and they need Medicaid, will I have to move out and sell the house before Medicaid will be approved? Is there any consideration that I'm living there?

Legal Matters

It always seems too early until it's too late. This slogan encourages all adults to record their wishes for future care while they still can. None of us knows when we might be too ill to direct our own care. With dementia, it's certain that we'll lose our capacity to choose the care we would want in the future. The sooner this critical task is completed, the better for all concerned.

Capacity is the ability to understand our options and to grasp the consequences of our choices. You don't have to remember who the president is to know you don't want to be kept alive artificially. A doctor can confirm that someone still has the capacity to make important decisions.

As with all adults, anyone with dementia needs a durable power of attorney, a medical power of attorney, an advance directive, and a will. Because all adults need these documents, I suggest not singling out the person with dementia to get this task done. Make it a family affair. Doing it together often eases a loved one's fear that they are somehow being taken advantage of.

Consulting an elder law attorney is important. Using an elder law attorney instead of the family attorney is like using a cardiologist instead of the family doctor. With dementia, you need a specialist. An elder law attorney will know the latest federal and state regulations.

Now is not a time for DIY documents downloaded from a website. You can use that type of service to start the process, but be sure an attorney reviews any paperwork before signing. I promise you that any funds you spend on an attorney will save more in money and anguish down the road.

Power-of-attorney documents may be durable or medical. You need both. A durable power of attorney allows the person named to conduct business on the signer's behalf. A medical power of attorney allows decisions on medical care, including choice of care providers and settings. Most people with dementia can be cared for with a durable and a medical power of attorney, but there are limits to these documents.

Having a power of attorney allows you to make decisions only when the signer cannot speak for themselves. A power of attorney cannot overrule the one who signed the document. If they want their drug-addicted nephew to take them to the bank every week, you can't stop them. That requires guardianship.

Guardianship is for someone who no longer understands their own actions but insists on making decisions for themselves.

Becoming a guardian involves going to court. The cost is usually in the thousands of dollars.

In court, you must prove that the person does not understand the effects of their choices and show who is best suited to be the guardian. The judge will decide on those two matters. The person with dementia has the right to be in the courtroom to hear all evidence and speak on their own behalf. They also have the right to bring an attorney. Once a guardian is appointed, it takes another trip to court to change it.

Not all families operate like an episode of *Little House on the Prairie*. Old rivalries and resentments often intensify under the stress of a dementia diagnosis. There may be competing interests for how assets are used for care. People do extreme things when money is involved. Protecting your loved one's interests requires legal action early on. Rest assured that whatever the situation is, attorneys have heard it all before.

WHAT TO SAY

- "Here's a news story about a 40-year-old woman who had a stroke. Her husband doesn't want life support for her." Pause to let that sink in. "I wouldn't want to be on life support if I were that sick. Would you?" Introduce the subject in a nonthreatening context.

- "I was thinking about what we said yesterday about what we'd want if we were really sick. What if you couldn't say what you wanted? Who would you want to speak for you?" This subject is too much for a single conversation. Approach it in bite-size pieces to prevent overwhelming your loved one or arousing suspicion about your motives.

- "I've never gotten around to making a will or an advance directive. I want to get that done. It's a lot to think about. Would you do it with me?" You want to normalize the process of getting legal documents in place as much as you can.

- Educate yourself on the recommended legal documents. Go to Alz.org and type "legal documents" in the search bar to find the Alzheimer's Association's thorough guide to legal matters.

- Find an elder law attorney by asking friends and family. Visit NAELA.org to search by zip code through the National Academy of Elder Law Attorneys. Some attorneys don't provide services for someone with a dementia diagnosis, so ask before making an appointment.

- To find local legal help for free or at a reduced cost, visit Lawhelp.org for a current listing of government and non-profit resources throughout the country.

- Look at an advance directive tailored for use in dementia care. A great example is at Dementia-directive.org. Look this form over before seeing an attorney to optimize the use of time when you do meet.

- Consider an initial meeting with an attorney without your loved one. If your loved one refuses to see an attorney or is questioning your motives, the attorney can advise you on next steps. You wouldn't be the first to have those problems.

- Try to schedule appointments that will involve your loved one at their best time of day. Many people are sharper in the morning than later in the day.

- Request a dated letter from the physician verifying that your loved one has the capacity to make important decisions. The closer the date of the letter to the date of legal documents, the better.

- Talk with your family in advance about the legal decisions that will need to be made. The more transparent the process of making decisions, the fewer chances of conflict later on.

- Consider enlisting the help of someone your loved one respects. A long-time friend, spiritual advisor, or clergy member may get further discussing a difficult topic than you can.

- What documents do you recommend for someone with dementia?

- How do you charge for your services? Hourly? A flat fee? Is there a discount for simultaneously preparing documents for two people (commonly spouses)?

- How can I best protect my loved one from fraud?

- What circumstances would lead you to recommend seeking guardianship?

- Are there legal ways to protect my loved one's assets if they ever need to apply for Medicaid?

- What are the laws on using a nanny cam to monitor care in my home or in a facility?

Long-Term Care

Sooner or later, almost all people with dementia will need some form of long-term care. This thought can be scary. There are many options to consider, and the media tell us horror stories about most of them.

Then there are the promises we made to always provide a loved one's care at home. Every family is different when it comes to who will help provide care. Notice I said "who *will* help," not "who *can* help." Not everyone is going to embrace the role of caregiver.

Dementia caregiving is a roller coaster that's hard to imagine at the start. As brain failure progresses, the physical and emotional demands on the caregiver escalate. We eventually must tap outside help if we expect to go the distance with our loved one.

The main types of long-term care are home health, adult day care, and full-time facility care. Each has its place over the years that dementia normally lasts.

HOME HEALTH

Home help with caregiving most often comes from a nurse's aide or a companion. Companions don't have to have formal training. They can supervise and engage someone who isn't safe alone. They can provide housekeeping, meal preparation, or transportation.

A certified nursing assistant (CNA) has completed 60 to 180 hours of classroom and clinical training and passed a state exam. CNAs care for people who can't perform activities of daily living without assistance. They can help with bathing, dressing, toileting, eating, and mobility.

Home help may be hired privately or through an agency. It's often tempting to hire privately because the cost is much lower than an agency charges. It also means that the person providing the care receives the amount you pay. At agencies, the person providing the care receives only a small portion of what you pay.

But hiring privately is risky business. It bypasses the safeguards that an agency provides, like routine criminal background checks, insurance against theft or other losses in your home, and workers' comp insurance. Nurse's aides have one of the highest rates of on-the-job back injuries. If an injury happens to a private caregiver, you could be on the hook for their medical care.

Hiring privately also means the Internal Revenue Service views you as an employer. You'll have to deal with taxes, Social Security, and unemployment payments if you want to stay legal. Despite these disadvantages, many people still use private caregivers. It's not a practice I recommend.

ADULT DAY CARE

Another option for long-term care is adult day care. These centers allow caregivers to continue working or to have breaks from the demands of care. It's best to ease a loved one into this new setting for partial days a few times a week. You can increase their hours from there. Some centers offer auxiliary services for an additional charge, like haircutting and bathing.

Many people will balk at going to the center with a hundred excuses. Call it going to work, to the club, to their volunteer job helping older people—whatever normalizes going. Expect that some days they'll hate it, and other days they'll love it. The primary benefits are the socialization and increased physical activity they can't get at home. Costs are also lower compared to in-home care.

FULL-TIME FACILITY CARE

When most people hear the term *long-term care*, they think of nursing homes or assisted-living facilities. But memory care is booming in the assisted-living industry. Most people with dementia can be cared for in a memory care center throughout their illness.

Around-the-clock care in a facility doesn't always mean a permanent move-in. Most facilities offer short stays for respite care. A respite stay allows primary caregivers time away from the demands of their role. Minimum stays apply, usually five to seven nights.

Most caregivers want to keep their loved one at home, but doing so is not always safe for either caregiver or care recipient. When home becomes unsafe, moving a loved one into a care facility is fraught with emotion. The head may understand the need, but the heart is a different story.

Fear and guilt are the primary feelings a caregiver will have over this transition. Will they really take care of her? What if he needs to go to the bathroom and no one's right there? What if she falls and no one knows? How do I know they won't abuse him?

Most dementia caregivers are plagued by guilt. If we're caring for a parent, we think of what they've given us through the years. A spouse's vows to be there in sickness and in health loom large. So, we want to be perfect. We want to ease our loved one's suffering. We lose perspective on what's realistic.

Now is a good time to remember that feelings are not facts. We may feel like placement means we've failed. That feeling is not a fact. Dementia is a phenomenon like nothing else we've seen. None of us is equipped to tackle it on our own. And safety must rule the day.

Families often ask me when it is time to move a loved one to facility care. My standard marker is safety for all involved: when a person with dementia is having falls; when a caregiver can no longer manage the care of a confused, combative loved one; when no one sleeps anymore; or when a loved one wanders after finding the one door accidentally left unlocked. These situations are unsafe.

Moving a loved one into memory care is not the end of caregiving. It simply relieves much of the physical burden of care. One thing it does enable is a return to the role of spouse or child or sibling. Years of caregiving can erase those roles, relegating us to being only a nurse. Full-time care by others allows us to be who we used to be to our loved one.

WHAT TO SAY

- "I know you do well on your own, but I would feel better knowing someone else was here." Take the focus off your loved one's needs when introducing home care. Highlight why help is needed for your sake. Framing the suggestion around your own needs makes it harder for them to refuse the care.

- "John, I'm going to lunch with my friend. Sarah is here if you need anything. I'll be back at two o'clock. I wrote it down for you." Use a whiteboard to list where you're going, who will help while you're gone, and what time you'll return.

- "I know it's hard to understand. But I'm just not strong enough to do everything you need to keep you safe." There's no easy way to allay your loved one's fears about full-time care in a facility. Keep explanations short. Use the broken-record technique. Keep repeating, "I'm just not strong enough to keep you safe."

- "I need to go now, but I'll be back soon." When first leaving a loved one in a care facility, enlist the help of the staff to make your exit. The harder you try to make it alright, the more upsetting it's likely to be for everyone.

WHAT TO DO

AT HOME AND DAY CARE

- Recognize that supplementing your care with professional caregivers is often in your loved one's best interests. You may think it's for your benefit, but ultimately it's for them.

- Ask friends and family for recommendations when you're looking for any long-term care.

- When starting home care, give your loved one a few short episodes of having another person in your home.

- Make a list of exactly what you want a caregiver to do while they're on duty. Tell them the list is to help both of you understand expectations. Make it clear to any agency you may use what you need the caregiver to do.

- Be specific in your expectations. Instead of "Keep Mom company," list a few activities she likes. Try "Read from one of the books on her table" or "Watch *Wheel of Fortune* with her."

- Keep your interactions with other caregivers at a professional level. Many problems can arise when an aide develops a false feeling of being "part of the family." You can be friendly but still maintain professional boundaries. They are in your home to help you and your loved one. You are not their social worker or confidant. Don't add their worries to your own.

- When workers don't meet your expectations, kindly let them know. Most of the time, it's because they weren't clear on what was or wasn't required.

- When starting with home care or day care, know that it's like your child's first day at school. They may protest when you leave, but two minutes later they're focused on something else.

AT A FULL-TIME FACILITY

- Begin looking at memory care options before you know you will need them.

- Do your research on facilities you want to consider. Every state has a website that provides information on past inspections of each facility. Check out at least a few of the resources at the end of this book (page 160). Use the experiences of others to guide you.

- Tour a care facility with your loved one while they can give you feedback. Tell them you want to see where they would be most comfortable if they're hospitalized and need more care before coming home.

- If your loved one doesn't accompany you for touring, ask another family member or close friend to go with you. Their second set of eyes and intuition are important.

- Beware of the fancy-schmancy facilities. The more money invested in physical assets, the less there is for hiring and training staff. This concern doesn't mean a place can't have both. Just be careful—not all that glit ters is gold.

- Ask to visit a prospective facility for a meal. Notice the food and presentation. Watch how the staff interact with the residents (industry lingo for those who live there).

- Notice the demeanor of the staff as you walk around the building. Are they smiling and friendly or nose down and busy?

- Pay attention to any odors encountered. Ask to see a current resident's bathroom. You're looking for cleanliness.

- Look at the posted calendar of resident activities. Notice if there are events off-site or only in-house. The best programs include off-site events to get residents outside and give them a change of scenery.

- Before you sign *any* service agreement, go over it with a fine-tooth comb. Sleep on it first. Would you buy a house without carefully reading the contract? Your loved one's well-being is way more important, so take your time. Have an attorney review anything you're not totally clear on.

- Red alert: Look for any mention of "binding arbitration" in an agreement. Strike it out. You should not have to keep this clause to admit your loved one. It means that if they kill your loved one, your only recourse is arbitration—you cannot sue them. If someone insists they won't accept your loved one without that condition, your best bet is to run to the next facility on your list.

WHAT TO ASK A PROSPECTIVE PROVIDER

QUESTIONS FOR ALL PROVIDERS

- What information do you obtain from potential staff before hiring them?

- What training have the staff had regarding people with dementia?

- How do the staff know what kinds of help my loved one needs?

- Will one or two aides provide care, or does the number depend on other factors?

- What services are covered under your base rate? Are there additional services available? What does each one cost?

ADDITIONAL QUESTIONS FOR HOME HEALTH AGENCIES

- Can your staff provide transportation? Would they use their car or mine? How is insurance guaranteed?

- How will your staff know we have cats/dogs/smoking in the house, in case of allergies?

- What kinds of things are staff not allowed to do while on duty?

- How many different caregivers will be assigned to our care?

- What should I do if I have a concern about my loved one's care?

- How does your billing work?

- What is your cancellation policy?

- What reasons would lead you to discharge my loved one from your care? How much notice would I receive?

- Do you accept Medicaid?

ADDITIONAL QUESTIONS FOR ADULT DAY CARE

- Can you describe how a typical day would go for my loved one?

- What should I do if I have a concern about my loved one's care?

- How does your billing work?

- What is your cancellation policy?

- What are reasons you would discharge my loved one from your care? How much notice would I receive?

- Do you accept Medicaid?

ADDITIONAL QUESTIONS FOR LONG-TERM CARE FACILITIES

- How many clients/residents is each aide caring for? Does that number change in the evening and overnight? Does the number change on the weekend?

- What is your staff turnover rate?

- Can you describe what a typical day would look like for my loved one? Are meals, wake-ups, and bedtime on a set schedule?

- What happens if my loved one doesn't eat? Can I bring in favorite foods for them? Can that food be stored just for them?

- What furniture and other belongings can we bring?

- How will I be kept informed of my loved one's condition?

- What services are covered under your base rate? Are there additional services available? What does each one cost?

- How is medical care managed? Are there a psychiatrist, podiatrist, and dentist that visit?

- Is transportation to appointments available? Is there an additional cost?

- Can I speak privately with a few staff members or family members?

- How many head nurses or directors have you had in the past three years? How many administrators have you had in that time? [Turnover in key positions can be a red flag. More than two in three years is worrisome.]

- What would I do if I had a concern about my loved one's care?

- How does your billing work?

- Do you accept Medicaid?

- What are your refund and transfer policies?

- What are reasons you would discharge my loved one? How much notice would I receive?

- Do you offer hospice care?

How Are You Doing?

Whew! Was this chapter heavy or what? You may be stunned by how much there is to think about. It's overwhelming if you look at all of it together. Staying sane means setting priorities and doing one thing at a time.

The emotions associated with prepping for the future will tempt you to delay. That temptation is normal. Find a willing friend or family member to help you stay on track. The quickest way to fail in dementia caregiving is trying to go it alone. I promise there's someone out there who wishes they had a way to help you.

Make yourself a calendar with the things you need to do. Use the "What to Do" for each topic to guide you. Share your calendar with your confidant. Ask them to check on your progress every week. Tell the truth when they ask. Share what seems to be holding you back from steps you know you need to take.

You hear a lot about taking care of yourself as a dementia caregiver. The term *self-care* often elicits thoughts of bubble baths, massages, and nights out with friends. Those opportunities are great when you can get them.

But self-care includes the little things you can do daily. Finding someone to keep you moving on your calendar counts. Saying no when you already have too much to do counts. Accepting "good enough" without guilt for missing "just right" counts. Remember that you don't have to go to a spa to treat yourself kindly.

CHAPTER SIX

END-OF-LIFE CARE

Henry walked the hospice nurse to her car and watched as she drove away. Before going back in the house, he stopped and looked across the adjoining fields to the farm he and Angelo had worked all these years.

Inside, Angelo was sleeping. The nurse had helped the certified nursing assistant (CNA) give him a good bath and put clean sheets on the bed. Sinking into the chair beside Angelo, Henry was glad for the fresh smell. Closing his eyes, he thought about the amazing people he'd met through hospice.

There was Joyce, the social worker who often appeared with her golden retriever Max in tow. This always drew a smile. Tony was the chaplain who visited once a week and heartened Henry with his prayers. There was Ann, the nurse, and Angelo's two CNAs, Laura and Beth. Henry was grateful for the love he saw when they cared for Angelo.

Looking back, Henry felt a little foolish that he'd fought using hospice services for so long. It had felt too soon. Things couldn't be that bad. It couldn't be the end. When he finally consented, it wasn't the end at all. It was the start. The start of a calmer, easier time for him to be with Angelo up until it was time for him to go. He only wished he'd agreed to hospice sooner.

End-of-Life Decisions

It always feels too soon until it's too late. Remember that slogan? A dementia diagnosis should spur any family to prepare their advance directives. The sooner, the better, while there's time for thoughtful discussion.

ADVANCE DIRECTIVE

An advance directive, sometimes called a living will, describes the care we would want near the end of life. It may also identify a medical power of attorney—the person we want to speak for us about our care if we can't speak for ourselves.

Self-determination is the principle behind an advance directive. It means that no one else has the right to choose our care as we approach our last days—not the child who has diligently cared for us, not the doctor, not even a beloved spouse of many years. We are master of our own fate.

Dementia creates unique considerations for the end-of-life care we would want. Many people have no medical conditions besides their dementia. They may live for years after they've lost cognitive awareness. But would they want to live in that condition?

An advance directive specific to people with dementia is important. It should allow care choices based on what stage of dementia a person is in, so that quality of life is a factor in making decisions. A great example of a dementia-tailored directive is available at Dementia-directive.org.

But what if it's too late? If your loved one doesn't already have an advance directive, what then? In the absence of an advance directive, a medical power of attorney is asked for decisions. When there isn't a medical power of attorney either, the next of kin is consulted.

Let's say someone didn't prepare any documents in advance. A doctor will want to talk to the legal next of kin. Laws defining who's considered next of kin vary from state to state. In most cases, the hierarchy goes from spouse to child to grandchild to parent to sibling to niece or nephew. The definition of spouse also varies among states.

When there's disagreement in the family about a loved one's care, the final decision belongs to the medical power of attorney. If no power of attorney is named, it goes to the next of kin.

Some family members will go to great lengths to gain the right to have the final say. Factors like preserving a potential inheritance and long-standing rivalries may be their motive. This situation can get sticky fast. If you're facing a similar scenario, get thee to an elder law attorney as soon as possible. You need accurate information on your options.

TYPES OF DECISIONS

What kinds of decisions might be needed for a loved one? The use of life support, cardiopulmonary resuscitation, feeding tubes, hospitalization, dialysis, life-prolonging medications, and hospice care are the most common issues. Options for each intervention range from doing nothing to doing everything humanly possible.

One challenge in making these decisions is the pressure you may face from others. This pressure may come from friends, family members, or medical professionals. Physicians are getting better in their approach, but many remain biased toward aggressive care. They don't always set aside their own experience and values.

Feeding tubes are an example. When swallowing is impaired, the doctor may offer placing a feeding tube. In dementia care, feeding tubes may make the doctor or the family feel better, but they do not extend life expectancy for those in advanced dementia. They only cause more suffering. In 2014, the American Geriatrics Society issued a position statement on the use of feeding tubes in advanced dementia. The society concluded that these tubes offer little to no benefit but increase the burden to the patient. You need this information because many doctors have yet to get the word.

Another truth to remember is that when a person is in a life-threatening situation, doctors often ask the wrong question of the family. They ask, "What do you want?" Well, what I want is for my loved one to have never had this terrible experience.

Doctors should be asking, "What do you believe your loved one would want?" This issue goes back to the principle of self-determination: It's not about what we want; it's about what they would want.

I often advise families to think about it this way: Imagine that for half an hour, your loved one could somehow return to being themselves. They could understand their situation and what their options are. What do you think they would say to do?

Suppose your loved one would say, "Leave me the heck alone and let me die in peace." What if that wish is different from what you want the doctors to do? As agonizing as it is, putting your loved one's wishes over your own is an enormous gift of love. We honor them as we sacrifice our wants for what's best for them.

WHAT TO SAY

- "Dad always said he didn't want to be kept alive on any machine." In the absence of an advance directive, there still may be comments or experiences of your loved one that can guide your decisions.

- "If I didn't know my family, I wouldn't want to try to keep living. Would you, Mom?" These discussions shouldn't be one-sided. Expressing your wishes can open the door to a loved one sharing theirs.

- "It's so awful when Jo goes to the emergency room. She doesn't know what's going on or who's going to do something to her next. I don't want her to go anymore." You can ask a doctor for a do-not-hospitalize order. This type of order especially helps if your loved one is in a facility. Facilities worry about liability and may send residents to the emergency room "just in case."

- "Uncle Bill has been on the ventilator for three days now. The doctor said if he didn't get better by now, he probably won't ever get better." Even if someone is already on life support, there are ways to discontinue that aggressive care and keep them comfortable in the process.

WHAT TO DO

- Talk with your loved one while they can still understand the conversation. Keep it simple. The more words you use, the harder it is for them to process and respond.

- Model how to express wishes for future care. Everyone will have to answer these questions someday.

- Talk with your family periodically about what your loved one might want for their end of life. Theoretical discussions every now and then can prepare you for reality down the road.

WHAT TO ASK YOUR DOCTOR

Prior to any test or procedure, ask these questions. Unless your loved one is in an immediate crisis, don't let people rush the process for you and your family

- What is this test or procedure for?

- How likely is it that we'll get the desired information or effect?

- How will the results change my loved one's care?

- How will this procedure affect their quality of life?

- If we agree to this treatment, how and when will we know if it is going to work?

- If we agree and then change our minds, how would that be handled?

- Do we have to give you an answer today?

Hospice

As a medical specialty, hospice is plagued by more mis-information than almost any other. Hospice care has changed dramatically in recent years. Lots of people still think that hospice care is for the deathbed. But that notion went out with lava lamps and corded phones.

Today, hospice is about quality of life for as long as a person may have left on earth. As medicine has advanced, people are living longer with terminal illnesses. As a result, hospice has expanded its focus from the last few days of life to months and even years of care.

Enrolling in hospice care requires a shift in our mindset. It requires letting go of medical treatment aimed at curing an illness. Its purpose is to make the best of whatever time is left, which means controlling difficult symptoms and promoting whatever the ill person values most in life.

Family education and support are also important parts of hospice care.

Hospice care is delivered by a team of professionals that includes a physician, nurses, nurse's aides, social workers, and chaplains. It may also include physical or occupational therapists and music therapists. All of these professionals are there to promote quality, not quantity, of life.

With dementia, it can be confusing to know if a loved one is ready for hospice. The normal requirement is a life expectancy of six months or less. In dementia, that window is almost impossible to identify. So, there is a different set of criteria for people with dementia.

For someone with dementia to qualify, they must be unable to walk, dress, or bathe on their own. They must be incontinent of bowel and bladder intermittently or always. Their speech must be mostly unintelligible.

Someone with dementia needs to meet those conditions *and* to have had one of the following within the past 12 months: aspiration pneumonia, pyelonephritis, septicemia, multiple bedsores at stage 3 or 4, fever returning after antibiotics, difficulty swallowing or refusing to eat, weight loss of more than 10 percent of their body weight, or a body mass index less than 18.

I know that's a lot of medical gobbledygook. I've spelled it out because not all doctors know the current criteria for hospice. Not all doctors are fans of hospice, feeling that they can provide the same care without it. So, your doctor may balk when you ask if it's time to consider hospice care.

If your doctor is resistant, you can call any local hospice provider and ask for an evaluation. Most have dealt with reluctant family doctors before. They'll visit you to hear about your loved one and see if they can help. It's much better to call before you need them than to delay the wonderful help they can provide.

Like everything else in health care, there are good providers and there are lousy providers. If you encounter a hospice lemon, don't hesitate to contact another provider. You can compare local hospices through Medicare.gov/hospicecompare. This site shows how long a hospice has been in business, whether it's nonprofit or for profit, how big it is, and more.

Gone are the days when calling in hospice meant giving up hope. We all need hope to live. With hospice, we hope for different things than we did before. We hope for moments of joy, of peace, of relationship. We hope for as many good days as we can get. And we hope for a peaceful time when we finally say goodbye.

- "I say we have another bowl of ice cream!" Now is the time to let your loved one have and do anything that brings them pleasure. If Uncle Jerry wants a cigarette, it's time to let him burn one down.

- "Pop is tired, Mom. I just don't think he would want to go through any more tests." Once your loved one develops choking problems, you know you're entering the most advanced stage. If a doctor suggests a swallowing test, ask what difference it will make in your loved one's comfort. *None* is the short answer.

- "Arthur, you know I've loved you from the first time we met. But it's time for you to let go. It's time for you to rest. I'll be okay. Gary and the girls will look out for me." Giving a loved one permission to leave this world is a great gift. We know that hearing is the last sense to fail. Their spirit is still in there. They will hear you.

WHAT TO DO

- Accept that hospice care is not just for the very end of life. It can breathe new life into any weary caregiver's soul.

- Call a local hospice provider and ask if they offer any education on what hospice is and how it works. It's better to learn about it in advance so you'll know what they can offer down the line.

- As your loved one's disease worsens, keep visits from friends or family short. It's still helpful for them to keep a routine with limited disruption.

- Let the hospice nurse's aides do the hardest tasks, like bathing and changing sheets. You want to be spouse, son, daughter, sibling, or friend as much as you can, leaving the nurse duties to someone else for a change.

- Take advantage of the respite hospice provides. Every three months, the Medicare hospice benefit pays for five nights of care in a facility. Take a break when you can; there are more exhausting days ahead.

- Say whatever you want to convey to your loved one. After attending hundreds of people in their last days and hours, I can promise you, they're no longer hearing with their diseased brain. They're hearing with their heart.

WHAT TO ASK YOUR DOCTOR

- When would you start to think about bringing in hospice?

- Is there a hospice provider you have had a good experience with?

- Would there be any harm in my talking with them well before we might need them?

- Could we go over my loved one's medications? I would like to know what benefit there is in continuing each one.

- How can we make sure my loved one receives only comfort measures?

- Can you explain why morphine is given near the end? How does that work?

How Are You Doing?

It doesn't matter how long your loved one has been sick. It doesn't matter that you've known all along that dementia is a terminal disease. It doesn't matter how many times you've rehearsed these conversations in your head. It doesn't matter. The bottom line is that now is a time of sorrow.

Your loved one is going to need you all the way through. To make it, you must use the relief time others give you by taking care of yourself. Trying to be a superhero may sound good in theory, but your body and your mind need rest. Not caring for yourself may seem like the easier way, but the toll self-neglect takes is never worth the price.

Lie down for half an hour without worrying whether you can fall asleep. Take a 10-minute walk outside. Soak in a tub until you look like a prune, knowing your loved one is being watched. Your loved one deserves the best care they can get, and so do you.

PART THREE

CARING FOR YOURSELF

CHAPTER SEVEN

HOW CAREGIVING AFFECTS YOU

JOSCELYN

Joscelyn stared at the woman in the mirror, wondering who she was. She knew she saw this woman every day when she brushed her teeth or did her hair. So, when did the woman become a stranger?

Joscelyn was 52 when her mother moved in with her. Mom had vascular dementia and wasn't safe to be alone anymore. Six years later, Joscelyn tried to remember when her own hair turned to more gray than brown. When did the extra chins appear? How had she given up on that woman in the mirror?

That question wasn't hard to answer. Her days started any- where between 4:00 a.m. and 9:00 a.m. From then until late night, it was all go, go, go. Getting mom to appointments, doing laundry, and grocery shopping. The list felt endless.

Looking back at the mirror, Joscelyn felt a twinge of resent- ment. None of her friends had the responsibilities she did. They weren't working full-time and coming home just in time to see the aide shoot out of the drive like a rocket. They didn't spend their entire weekend doing a thousand chores.

Then there were her siblings. They bragged on Facebook with vacation pictures, new landscaping for the house, a child's birthday party. But not one had spent more than half an hour at a time with their mother in the past two years.

The Emotional and Physical Toll

The fear brought on by a loved one's dementia diagnosis is staggering. We're on a bus ride down a congested street, and there's no driver at the wheel. Here's where we say that if you aren't freaking out, you clearly don't understand the situation. The future looms large. The most dire scenes play through our minds. We hardly know where to start.

Much of our fear comes from feeling like we're totally unprepared to take on the task ahead. Most of the time, we *are* totally unprepared. Have you ever watched someone else walk through dementia caregiving? Probably not

For most of us, we're in foreign territory. What reference point do we have for helping someone live with dementia? Had you even heard of dementia before 10 years ago? Not many of us planned on being trailblazers at this stage of our lives.

I like to remind people that dementia caregiving is a voluntary job. As harsh as it sounds, we always have the right to walk away. Nobody *has* to do anything. We may feel like we have no choice in the matter. But feelings aren't facts. The fact is we all have the right to say no.

I just want you to remember that there are other options. If it ever becomes too much, you don't have to sacrifice yourself in the process. What is the value of the rescuer going down with the one in danger? Not to mention that you deserve to survive with a shred of sanity still intact.

We caregivers are notorious for ignoring our own needs until we're forced to take care of them. We go without sleep. We eat too much junk food or forget to eat at all. We don't have time to exercise. We isolate ourselves because no one understands us anyway. We foster these habits at our own peril—and that of our loved one.

The reality is that none of us is superhuman. We can get away with burning the candle at both ends for a while. But sooner or later, the wick runs out and we get burned. Remember that dementia caregiving normally lasts for years, not weeks or months. If we want to keep going, we have to accept help whether we like it or not.

The first help I recommend for all caregivers is professional counseling or therapy. If you got hit by a bus, would you say no to medical care because you thought you could handle it? Yet, when we are broadsided by the emotional bus of dementia, we expect to patch things together without professional help. There is no time to worry about looking weak or whether a stranger really can help you. Your loved one needs you sane. Therapy goes a long way in meeting that goal.

The other help no caregiver should go without is connecting with other dementia caregivers. Knowing you're not alone, that nobody has this thing figured out, that we're all just doing the best we know how is invaluable. Whether it's a face-to-face support group or an online group or both, being kind to yourself includes joining in. I've listed some support group resources in the back of the book (page 163). Now, let's look at some of the wheels on that emotional bus I mentioned a moment ago.

STRESS AND ANXIETY

Stress and anxiety are daily companions for most us. What's coming next? When will I have to stop working? How am I going to take care of Mom and handle three teenagers at the same time? Am I doing this right? Are they getting the right care?

Stress does terrible things to our bodies. It messes with our immune system, wrecks our sleep, raises our blood pressure, and gives us headaches, chest pains, and stomach problems. We aren't built to live this way unceasingly.

Although we can't eliminate the hamster wheel in our minds, we can learn to slow that thing down. Physical activity, scheduled time away from caregiving, learning to say no, breathing exercises, keeping a journal, eating healthy food, and talking with a counselor are all good tools. Taming stress and anxiety takes action on our part. They rarely get better on their own.

FRUSTRATION AND ANGER

Frustration and anger are seldom far behind our stress and anxiety. Heaven knows there's plenty to be frustrated about: answering the same question four times in five minutes, being told no when you ask another family member for help, doctors who don't return phone calls, disappearing friends, loved ones who say they don't need to go to the bathroom right before they pee all over the carpet, and so on.

Then there are the cosmic questions. Why did this have to happen to Grandma? What about Roger's dreams for these years of our lives? Why do people have to suffer like this? The list goes on and on.

Many of us have been socialized to believe that anger is something nice people don't express, that being angry indicates some flaw in our character. As a dementia caregiver, you will feel anger; sometimes, lots of anger.

Denying angry feelings or berating ourselves for having them only makes it worse. At times, our anger is an effort to keep the depths of our sadness at bay. Justifiable anger often hurts less than acknowledging our bone-crushing sorrow.

SADNESS AND DEPRESSION

How could anyone watch someone they love struggle with a terminal illness without feeling deep sadness? Sorrow and grief become constant companions as we experience losses both big and small. Dementia has been called "the long goodbye" for a reason.

Anticipatory grief is also a part of the caregiver's journey. We know how the story ends from the day we hear a dementia diagnosis. We try not to dwell on our loved one's demise, but that reality bubbles just below the surface of our everyday lives.

Although deep sadness is a normal response to the circumstances we face, clinical depression is not. Recognizing where normal sadness stops and depression begins is often hard to see in ourselves.

If we escape depression during our caregiver journey, we are the exception and not the rule. Depression creeps up on us. It can have us in a chokehold before we even see it coming. You aren't losing your mind. You're just depressed.

Signs to watch for include insomnia, trouble concentrating, weight loss, and weight gain. Increased alcohol or medication use may be a sign of depression. Losing interest in hobbies or other things that used to be enjoyable is another clue. Feelings of hopelessness loom, and self-esteem is at rock bottom.

We don't want to go out. We don't want to talk to anyone. And we're so exhausted that it hurts to breathe. Headaches, flare-ups of other chronic illnesses, and a big, fat zero in the libido department are physical signs of depression. If you think you might have depression, you probably do.

GUILT

Do you ever feel like if you're breathing, you're probably doing it all wrong? Welcome to guilt on a scale you may have never felt before. Being your own worst enemy isn't just an old saying in the world of dementia care.

Dementia caregiving doesn't come with a manual. There are no magic formulas. It's like raising kids: You make it up as you go along. But our expectations of ourselves can be astronomical, mostly because we want with all our hearts to do it well.

We long to take away the pain for ourselves and for our loved one. When we find that we can't, we assume it's because we're doing something wrong. If only we were more patient, more knowledgeable, more assertive, less assertive, happier to care for our loved one—and on it goes—then it would be alright. But we aren't, which makes us feel guilty.

Few traumas evoke such feelings of guilt as when we have to place a loved one in full-time facility care. The dangers of frequent falls, uncontrolled rages, or wandering every chance they get may give justification to our heads. Our hearts are a whole other ballgame. You'll likely feel guilty a lot. Feeling guilty doesn't mean you are guilty.

EXHAUSTION AND PHYSICAL ISSUES

In dementia caregiving, mental and physical exhaustion can quickly surpass anything you've ever felt before. Months and years on end of interrupted sleep, being responsible for all the duties of a household, and the physical demands of care-taking are enough to finish off Superman by lunchtime—no kryptonite needed.

Sustained stress and anxiety exact a terrible physical toll, and most of us caregivers are not exactly young. Throw in menopause or its male equivalent, chronic illness, or even the common cold, and it can yield disaster. And who will care for our loved one if we go down?

Even when we're supposedly sleeping, we have an ear out for any sign of trouble. The least little bump in the night, and we're up and in full-on battle mode. Our bodies aren't designed to stay in fight-or-flight mode at all times.

When we're weighed down with all the tasks allotted to us, it's easy to slide on picking up our own prescriptions. Keeping that follow-up appointment with the cardiologist seems like too much trouble. And rest? Well, we'll rest when this is all over. But then it isn't over, and we're in trouble.

Taking care of our body, our soul, and our mind is the only way to be the best caregiver we can possibly be. Doctors, thera-pists, willing friends, or family can help. Cast your net wide from the very beginning to yield the best results.

- How do I know what normal anger in this situation looks like?

- Is it possible I have depression?

- Is there anything I can do about my depression?

- Is there anything I can do about my anxiety?

- Are there any therapists you can recommend?

- Are there medications that can help any of these issues? (See the "Questions to Ask About All Medications" sidebar on page 38 for additional medication questions.)

Grief and Loss

Grief and loss rumble through our caregiving days with painful regularity. They begin before or at the time we hear a dementia diagnosis. Our grief gradually rises with each new stage of our loved one's disease.

Anticipatory grief, grieving for what we know is coming, is an unavoidable part of dementia caregiving. We all know where dementia leads. We know the last chapter is already written, and we're powerless to change it. Knowing our loved one will not survive triggers anticipatory grief. Knowing the losses they'll endure along the way also creates this type of grief.

The losses caused by dementia aren't as clear as a loss by death. When someone dies, we know when it happened. We know how it happened. We take part in certain rituals to mark the event. Our sorrow is understood by others who offer condolences and support.

Those things don't happen with the slow but inevitable losses of dementia. What we experience is called ambiguous loss. Ambiguous loss and the subsequent grief can come from two scenarios. Either someone is physically absent but emotionally present or they're physically present but emotionally absent. They're here, but they aren't here.

Ambiguous loss can cause our grief to freeze. Our grief is all dressed up but there's no place to go. We don't want to burden others, and they wouldn't understand, anyway. We can't pinpoint when the losses happened. We may feel silly for the moments that break our hearts.

It's easy to see the big triggers of feelings of grief and loss. Mourning is most intense at the time of diagnosis, at the time of moving a loved one into full-time care, and at the time of death. The losses that cause ambiguous grief may be big or small.

Some of the losses we experience are big enough to be easily recognized: plans for the future with a spouse, independence when our loved one can no longer stay at home alone, a job we love, companionship in our home.

But the little things may catch us by surprise and threaten to bury us in sorrow. Mom can't handle the trip to the hairdresser that happened every Friday for the past 30 years. Dad holds the toothbrush but has no idea what to do with it. Your partner can no longer drive wherever the two of you go. Your sibling has their first episode of incontinence and is mortified.

At some point, you may begin to wish for your loved one's suffering to end and for your six-ton burden to disappear. But the only way for that to happen is for your loved one to die. You're shocked to be daydreaming about your loved one's demise. It's called being human.

Any caregiver who says they never wish their loved one would die sooner rather than later is either in denial or lying. This thought is not shameful. Why would wishing your loved one to be free of dementia ever be anything but an act of deep love? Yet we beat ourselves senseless for thinking that way.

Watching a loved one decline from dementia has been called "the long goodbye." The danger of this mindset is it can prevent us from recognizing all that still remains. If we focus our attention solely on what is lost, we intensify our grief beyond what we would otherwise experience.

Dealing with grief and loss in dementia care requires a two-pronged approach. First, we need to recognize, acknowledge, and give voice to our grief. Second, we need to understand that all is not lost, that our loved one still has meaningful moments ahead, and that we must pay attention or we'll miss them.

Living one day at a time is the only way to survive dementia caregiving. Other answers to our grief are talking with others about our sorrow, being kind to ourselves for we are all fragile beneath our bravado, and seeking talk therapy with a professional. Taking regular breaks from caregiving gives us room to breathe as we grieve. Talking with clergy or other spiritual advisors allows us to ask our cosmic questions.

We may not be able to hope for a cure for our loved one. But we learn to hope for other things: for more good days than bad days, for a loved one's smile, for moments of lucidity coming out of the blue. And yes, we're allowed to hope for brighter days when this journey is over.

WHAT TO ASK YOUR THERAPIST, RELIGIOUS LEADER, OR TRUSTED FRIEND

- Why did my loved one have to get this disease?

- What kind of suffering is this? What are we supposed to do with it? What is its purpose?

- How can I love and hate my loved one at the same time?

- How can I want them here and wish them gone at the same time?

How Are You Doing?

These pages are painful to get through, aren't they? Give yourself a pat on the back. It takes courage to look at what's happening in your heart and mind right now.

I know I talked about living one day at a time. But the truth is that one day can often be way too much to consider all at once. Break your day down into hours. Getting through one hour at a time can be more manageable.

In the morning, think about what you hope the day will bring—appointments, housework, grocery shopping, the dreaded shower. Then stop each hour and think, "What's the next right thing for me to do right now?"

I'm not talking about baby steps here. I am talking about itty-bitty steps. If five minutes at a time is all you can hang on for, then five minutes at a time it is. I know that you can do it.

One way to stay present in today is to do a body scan. This mindfulness method is a way of connecting with the here and now. You can do an online search for "body scan" to find audio guides. I've listed some in the Resources section at the end of the book (page 160). What feels weird in the beginning can eventually provide sweet relief if you practice.

CHAPTER EIGHT

WORK-LIFE BALANCE

PHYLLIS

Phyllis slipped past the front desk and into her office, hoping no one would notice. For the second time this week, she was late. It wasn't her fault. She couldn't help that Mom had needed 30 minutes in the bathroom just as they were about to leave for day care.

But here she was. Her boss, Sylvia, had already given her one written warning. Chances were she would get another today. Sylvia had advised her to think hard before continuing to work when she couldn't manage it. "You don't want to ruin your good record here."

"How's your mama doing? I hope she's getting better."

The shrill voice sliced through Phyllis's reverie. Tammy's well-meaning inquiry grated on her nerves. It was all she could do not to snap back, "Hello? She has Lewy body, remember? Nobody with Lewy body dementia ever gets better! Their mind just goes further and further away until it's gone. And then they die. Get it?"

But Phyllis held her tongue. She knew Tammy meant well. God knows she wasn't the first person to be clueless about what Phyllis was going through. She mumbled something about Mom holding her own and headed for another cup of coffee. If she hurried, by lunchtime she could finish the report due yesterday.

Balancing Work and Caregiving

Whether we work full-time or part-time, our work matters to us for many reasons. Financial security is the obvious one. I'm fond of eating and having a roof over my head, so a paycheck is good for me. But work can also meet our needs for socialization and feelings of competence.

For dementia caregivers, the income from employment can be crucial. On average, caregivers spend over $5,500 a year on out-of-pocket care expenses. Copays, prescriptions, incontinence supplies, and paid caregiving help are only the start.

Not everyone has a spare $500 a month lying around. Work is often a necessity. Other benefits, like health insurance, retirement accounts, and paid time off, also matter. Working now can affect our income in the future, too.

The average American caregiver is 48 to 50 years old—peak earning time for most workers. Peak earnings history determines our monthly Social Security payments in retirement. Stepping down or out of the workforce entirely can diminish our peak earnings, decreasing our future income.

Work has important nonmonetary benefits. It can be a welcome relief from caregiving burdens. Work is a place for adult conversation, something often missing at home. Feelings of competence and pride in a job well done at work are hard to come by in the messy world of dementia care. A paycheck or a supervisor's compliment confirms that we are valuable to others.

Giving up the financial and emotional benefits of working outside the home is a difficult decision for anyone. It pays to have all the facts before deciding. You'll want to know about federal and state laws that protect family caregivers. And you'll want to know if you can receive pay for the care you give.

In 1993, the Family and Medical Leave Act (FMLA) went on the federal law books. The FMLA says that employers must allow up to 12 weeks of unpaid leave to care for a parent, spouse, or child. The employee remains on benefit plans and their position is secure, but there are important conditions and limitations to the FMLA.

The FMLA applies only to employers with 50 or more employees. About half of businesses in the United States fall below that size. For an employee to use the FMLA, they must have worked at least 1,250 hours in the past 12 months. The FMLA does not apply to caregiving for in-laws, siblings, or grandparents.

The Americans with Disabilities Act (ADA) offers some protection for caregivers. The ADA protects people with disabilities from discrimination or retaliation for needing time off work for medical reasons. It also provides the same protections for caregivers of people with disabilities. If you're passed over for a promotion or given a rotten schedule because of your work absences, you may have a claim against your employer.

Beyond federal protections, most states have laws to benefit caregivers. Because these laws vary widely by state, you'll want to consult a local attorney for the most accurate information. You should also do an online search for the subject "caregiver laws" for your state.

Many states now have programs that allow family caregivers to be paid for their time. The state's risk for fraud is high, so there's plenty of red tape to navigate. Local departments of social services, attorneys, or area boards for aging may provide help with the process.

WHAT TO DO

- Plan ahead for any conversation you want to have with your manager or the human resources department. Have a few options in mind that might help you, like working remotely or going to part-time work. Decide in advance how much information you want to disclose about your loved one's condition.

- Spend a few minutes before the meeting letting go of any negative emotions you're mired in at the moment. Lock yourself in the restroom to close your eyes and take six slow, deep breaths. Look in the mirror and remind yourself, "You've got this."

- Start off these discussions by confirming your commitment to the company and to the job.

- Offer a few ideas for changes to your work schedule, and be open to ideas the company may have. It's risky going into a meeting with only one acceptable outcome in mind.

- Maintain a professional approach in the meeting. Do your best to check your emotions at the door. You can express them later in a more appropriate setting.

- If you feel yourself on the verge of crying, take a moment to recompose before moving ahead. Don't beat yourself up if a few hot tears escape. We're only human.

WHAT TO ASK YOUR MANAGER OR HUMAN RESOURCES DEPARTMENT

- Where can I find the company's policies on taking leave? (You want a hard copy to read later, when you can concentrate on the details.)

- Is working remotely an option for any of my duties?

- Is it possible to vary my schedule to meet my commitments to the company and to my family?

- Are part-time hours a possibility?

- Is early retirement an option for me?

- How does the FMLA work here? What would I need to do to use it? Would that affect my health insurance or my retirement fund?

Arranging Outside Services

Accepting that we can't do it all ourselves is hard for many of us. The irony is that the more we insist on doing it all, the less effective we may become at doing any of it. To avoid letting down our loved one, the rest of the family, or our coworkers, arranging outside services may be key.

Think about the tasks that you hate the most or that are the biggest time drain. In our gig economy, there is often someone out there who can fill the bill. Housekeeping, laundry, meal preparation, lawn care, ferrying the kids around town, and shopping can all be hired out.

Finding help is a challenge we'll need to persevere through. Asking friends and family for recommendations is a great place to start. Many online sites list task-oriented services offered in most areas. Don't forget the community-services boards that many stores and restaurants maintain.

Arranging outside services doesn't always mean hiring someone. Friends or family may want to help but are unsure of what we need. Letting faith communities or other organizations we belong to know our needs can save important dollars for other expenses. Bartering with a friend is another way to keep costs down.

Friends or family who live too far to visit but want to help can be tapped to fund a cleaning service or order a meal for delivery from a restaurant local to you. Use your imagination in what would help you, and make those needs known.

- "Here's a list of things that would help me out. Is there something on it that you could do?" Have a list handy for when others say, "Call me if you need anything."

- "I know you prefer that I do these things, but I'm just one person. I'd rather spend time with you than do all these other things." Know that having outside help can be an adjustment for everyone in the household.

WHAT TO DO

- Sit down and make a list of all the things you can think of that need to be done on a regular basis. Identify which ones you hate the most or which ones take the most time and energy.

- Ask friends and family for recommendations of providers for the services you would rather delegate to someone else.

WHAT TO ASK PROSPECTIVE SERVICE PROVIDERS

- What services are covered under your base rate? Are there additional services available? What does each one cost?

- Are you bonded and insured?

- Can you provide references from others you have worked for?

- How does your billing work?

- What is your cancellation policy?

How Are You Doing?

Juggling work, caregiving, and other roles, like spouse or parent, is difficult and exhausting. When it's dementia caregiving in particular, it's enough to make anybody's head spin.

Here's a quick fix to change your focus after a stressful situation. Watch something funny. I'm not joking. Laughter increases blood flow to our brains, fires up and then cools down our fight-or-flight response for a relaxed feeling, and releases endorphins.

It can be hard to think of anything funny when you're in the middle of a meltdown. Enter the modern marvel known as online videos! Search for funny animals, funny kids, or funny grannies. You can even search for funny idiots—no short supply there. Just find something to squeeze out a few good belly laughs.

CHAPTER NINE

STAYING HEALTHY AND RESILIENT

ROSE

Rose rolled over and looked at the clock: 9:00 a.m.? That couldn't be right. She jumped up and checked her phone. Yep, it was 9:00 a.m., alright. A miracle.

Rose hadn't slept past 6:00 a.m. for the past two years. Every night, she slept with one eye half open and an ear tuned to hear if Bernadette was on the move. Since her sister had moved in two years ago, Rose had experienced extreme exhaustion.

Bernadette was up and down like a yo-yo most nights. She had no sense of day and night. Rose had hung on as long as she could. After a serious error at work, she was finally willing to do something about her lack of sleep.

Tiptoeing down the stairs, Rose peeked to see her sister and the home health aide, who had spent the night. The aide was showing Bernadette funny animal videos on her tablet. Wait! What was this?

Could it be? Yes, it was true! There sat Bernadette, and for the first time in six days, she was wearing a clean shirt. "I might live after all," mused Rose as she headed upstairs for some stretching and breathing exercises. She was excited to try out what she'd learned in yoga class last night.

Get Moving

Our human bodies are built to move. Why else would they come equipped with over 700 muscles and 300 joints? Our bodies get sluggish when we don't move enough. Lack of movement leads to stiffness and nagging aches and pains. Have you ever said "ouch" when getting up from a chair?

The benefits of exercise are numerous. Exercise lifts mood, improves heart health, and delays the muscle loss that comes with aging. It helps us sleep better, move better, and hurt less.

Exercise provides a concentrated dose of motion, but it's not the only way to get moving. Increasing your overall physical movement throughout the day may be more manageable than a 5K run. And it can do you a lot of good.

Most caregivers go all day doing for others, feeling like they don't have a moment to take care of themselves. If anyone has earned the right to take a break, you have. But sitting beyond a needed rest period will make you feel worse. There's a solution to this conundrum. Moving your body will make you feel better, and it's something you can do just yourself.

Here's the mental twist that will let you consider moving just for the sake of moving: When you choose moments of movement for no one's benefit but your own, it becomes a little reward for your body, something you deserve.

You can accomplish moving for the sake of moving in just a few minutes at a time. You can squeeze it in at unexpected moments. It costs nothing, and you don't need to find a caregiver sub for your loved one to accomplish and enjoy this kind of physical activity.

When you find yourself annoyed with someone or something, you can shift gears by thinking, "I'm going outside to do ten jumping jacks!" Those little moments will be your reward as you do something for you and only you. (The truth is, by rewarding yourself with movement, your loved one will get the benefit of a more energized, less stressed caregiver.) The more you move and the more parts of your body you move, the better you'll feel.

For some, concentrated activity in the form of exercise works best. You may regain your sanity while working your muscles at the gym, in a yoga class, or on the forgotten elliptical waiting for you downstairs. If you're one of those people, go ahead and engage in dedicated exercise.

But if you're not, try moving for the sake of moving. Shake a leg in the morning, reach for the ceiling after lunch, jump up and down before dinner, and do anything and everything that gets your muscles, tendons, and ligaments moving and stretching. Your commitment to engaging regularly in activity you enjoy will satisfy what your body needs. Doing good for your body will do good for your spirit, too.

WHAT TO DO

- Start small. A five-minute walk is a great beginning.

- Learn half a dozen stretches you can do at any point in the day. You can stretch in bed, in the shower, or from a chair. A few minutes of stretching a few times a day makes a big difference over time.

- Let technology help. A virtual assistant can talk you through all kinds of routines from 5 to 60 minutes at a time. Do an online search for fitness apps to find everything from abdomen exercises to line dancing.

- Find a friend to hold you accountable for keeping up. You may be on opposite sides of the world but can sweat in rhythm.

- Take advantage of community pools, which are usually inexpensive compared to gym memberships. Movement in water protects your joints and soothes the savage beast.

- How much physical activity do you recommend for me?

- Are there any limits I should consider when exercising?

- Are there any types of exercise I should avoid?

Eat Right

Food, glorious food! Food can boost our immune system, improve our mood, and lower our risk for dementia, cancer, stroke, and heart disease. It can also wreck our immune system, bomb our mood, and increase our risk for dementia, cancer, stroke, and heart disease. It's all about our choices.

Food affects what we feel mentally and physically. It affects our loved ones the same way. If there were a pill that could give the boost we feel when eating right, most of us would rush to be first in line.

Being the best caregiver you can be requires that you eat healthy. A nutritious diet means more fruits and veggies, fewer prepackaged processed foods, and limited sugar and fat.

Prepackaged processed foods are tempting when you're short on time for cooking. Sugar and high-fat comfort foods can be a trap for emotional eating. We feel down or stressed. We eat these foods, which give us immediate satisfaction. The foods then react with our bodies to make us feel more down or stressed. And the cycle repeats.

As with any change in habits, starting small will improve your chances for success. Setting a goal to eat like a trained athlete by the weekend leads to failure. Make one better choice each day, or choose an area to focus on each week.

Hydration is another biggie for how we feel mentally and physically. Our cells function best in a water-based environment.

When we fail to replenish that environment with fluids, we feel it. The good news is that when we do keep up our fluid intake, we feel the benefits.

WHAT TO DO

- Commit to making one change every one to two weeks. Examples are drinking 40 ounces of fluids (that aren't soda) each day, cutting sugar in half, and eating at least one salad or green leafy vegetable each day. You can build a lot of healthy habits over time.

- Ask a friend to join you and hold each other accountable.

- Find a store that lets you order groceries online for pickup or delivery. Some provide delivery for free. Even if you have to pay $5, the cost of poor food choices is much greater. Shopping from home with your feet up fosters better choices than the harried environment of a store.

- Search "easy healthy meals" online. You'll find ideas there to last until the cows come home.

- Keep a food diary for a week. Pay attention not only to what you eat but also to the times you eat:

  - Are there times when you forget meals? How long did you go before recharging with nourishment?

  - Did you stop eating at least two hours before bedtime for the sake of digestion?

- Are there any particular eating plans you would recommend?

- Should I focus on weight, cholesterol, or both?

- What actions would you recommend I take?

- Would you recommend I see a nutritionist? What goals would you suggest I set for working with them?

- Are there any supplements you would advise me to take?

Stay Connected

Finding safety in numbers holds especially true for dementia caregivers. Loneliness runs rampant among caregivers. It's easy to lose our way without mooring to other adults. We must widen our inner circle to have as many listening ears as possible. We're going to need them.

Unfortunately, there's no diagnosis that makes people disappear faster than dementia does. The level of ignorance about it in the general public is staggering, and people will avoid what they don't understand.

Every day, I hear from at least one dementia caregiver with disappearing friends and family. Friends are suddenly always busy. The community center your loved one attended and volunteered at for 20 years goes silent. Family members lamely cry, "I can't stand seeing them that way!" As if it were easy for you.

Other people's tendency to shy away is not something you have to take lying down. You can't control their actions, but you can influence them. You educated yourself about dementia. Educate those in your circle of family and friends, too. The more they understand, the less avoidance you may see.

Dwelling on the failure of others to act like they care is a trap. Searching for what you could say or do to make them straighten up is often a dead-end road. The emotional energy that search requires is better spent on things we can change.

You can share information about your loved one's current condition. You can express how much their involvement would mean. You can give them ideas for practical ways to help.

WHAT TO DO

- When people say, "Call me if you need anything," tell them that it would help if they called you on a schedule you choose to see what current needs are.

- When you first tell family and friends about the diagnosis, tell them how you feel about managing your loved one's care in the future.

- Give them a way to learn more about dementia and about caregiving. Copy the list of resources in the back of this book (pags 160–163). Print an article you found helpful.

- Ask those around you how they might be able to help when additional care is needed. Asking in advance allows for calm discussion before a crisis, when emotions run high.

- Find one or two people you can count on and set up a plan for regular communication, whether it's lunch once or twice a month, a 30-minute phone call on a set evening, a text each morning, or an e-mail exchange.

- If you or your loved one is part of a spiritual or other type of community, share the diagnosis with the leader. Express any concerns about being forgotten by them.

- Track how often you talk with someone other than your loved one about something other than your loved one.

Tick it off on your calendar if that helps. Commit to calling someone if it has been more than three days since you had an outside conversation.

WHAT TO ASK YOUR FAMILY AND FRIENDS

- Is there a morning when you could visit? (Let others know the best time of day for engaging your loved one and you.)

- Can we talk about something else? (Check yourself to avoid talking about nothing but your loved one. Set yourself a limit, such as allowing 10 minutes on the topic. We all need occasional reminders that the rest of the world still exists.)

- When can you come sit with Joe for two hours? (Ask directly for what you need. Thinking it's obvious what we need doesn't make it so.)

Support Groups

Other dementia caregivers are often the only ones who fully grasp what our life is like. When going through hard times, nobody wants to be judged. We especially don't need people who haven't done what we're doing to tell us what to do and how to feel.

What we need is someone to listen and to respond: *Me, too. That's so hard. This is what helped me.* Support groups created for dementia caregivers can provide this kind of understanding.

Support groups may be face-to-face or online. You can tap associations for specific brain diseases to find face-to-face groups in your area. You'll find a list of these in the Resources section at the end of this book (page 160).

Online support groups provide a place to go when you can't go anywhere. Facebook has many groups focused on different types of dementia. You're almost sure to find someone online at any hour of day or night, with members from around the globe. These groups are usually closed, which means only group members can see posts and comments. This restriction allows members to avoid any prying eyes of friends or family.

Memory cafés aren't support groups in the formal sense but provide great informal support. These social groups meet regularly. They provide people living with dementia and their caregivers a chance to relax and socialize with others who understand their situation. The Memory Cafe Directory website lets you search for groups in your area (see Resources, page 163).

Joining any support group can cause a bit of social anxiety. What will the other caregivers be like? What will we talk about? What if there are attention seekers or consistently negative people in the group? What will I sound like when I am there? What will the group think about me?

Groups tend to have their own approaches and flavors. Some are lighthearted, some are mostly educational, and some are a melting pot of many perspectives. To benefit from any group, you need to be comfortable there. You may want to belong to more than one group. You may try a group and feel it's not the one for you. Search for a sense of acceptance; you'll be glad you did.

WHAT TO DO

- Refer to the Resources (page 160) for how to locate groups in your area.

- Contact the group leader before your first meeting to hear a little about the group and how it functions.

- Give a group at least two meetings to decide if it's for you. You can't know if your first meeting was typical or a one-off session.

- Consider bringing a friend or family member with you. The extra support never hurts.

- If there's no memory café in your area, consider starting one. The Memory Cafe Directory has practical information on how to go about it.

- Take a look at some of the online support groups listed in the Resources (page 160). You won't be able to see posts without joining, but you can see each group's description of its focus.

- Does anyone else's loved one do this? (You don't have to feel alone. Whatever you're facing, there are others who can say, "Me, too.")

- Do you like your doctor/home health agency/day care center/memory care facility?

- Does anyone have family members who don't lift a finger to help but have plenty to say about what you're doing wrong? (I promise you this theme is common among caregivers.)

- How did you decide it was time to move your loved one into memory care?

- Do you ever feel like if your loved one doesn't take a shower soon, you're going to strap them on the hood of the car and head to the car wash? (Caregivers need a place to share all their thoughts without judgment. So much of caregiving is a laugh-or-cry proposition. It feels good to be with people who understand the value of both.)

- What do you do when all you want to do is drive away and never come back?

Be Kind to Yourself

Being kind to ourselves is a novel idea for many caregivers. Our expectations of ourselves often far outstrip what is humanly possible. Yet we berate ourselves when we feel we've made a wrong move.

Oh, dear reader, I wish I could reach out to give you a bear hug and invite you to literally cry on my shoulder for as long as you need. How easy it is to become our own worst critic in this thing called caregiving.

We indulge in self-criticism at our own peril and that of our loved one. One of the essential factors for quality of life in someone with dementia is the emotional stability of their primary caregiver. Our loved one deserves kindness, and so do we.

Being kind to yourself involves knowing and honoring your limits. I promise you have some. We may feel like we have no options, but feeling that way doesn't make it a fact. If your survival hinges on leaving for good, you have the right to take the person you care for someplace safe, and then go.

This notion of having options is especially important to those who haven't had a good past with the person needing care. There are plenty of parents who have been abusers all their lives, spouses who regularly drank up the rent money and blamed their husband or wife, and on and on the list of scenarios goes.

Being kind to yourself is a mix of small measures each day and large decisions as your loved one's disease progresses. Taking care of yourself comes in many forms. Self-care doesn't have to be big or expensive.

Saying no to someone can be an act of kindness to yourself. Arranging respite time away from caregiving is an act of kindness to yourself. So is managing your self-talk. Reading this book, and using some of its tips, is an act of kindness to yourself.

If you want to go the distance in your loved one's journey, being kind to yourself isn't optional; it's absolutely required. To be the best caregiver you can possibly be, you must respond on the many days when you're the one who needs your love the most.

- Make a list of things you love: things to do and things to hear, see, taste, and touch. Commit to making sure you indulge in at least one of them daily.

- Find a way to relax that works for you. Is it yoga, reading a book, returning to a forgotten hobby? Look for something you can spend a bit of time on every day.

- Learn mindfulness meditation. This practice isn't about lighting incense and chanting "om." It's a proven method of stress reduction that anyone can do. Search online for "mindfulness-based stress reduction" in your area to find classes near you. The Resources section (page 160) includes a website where you can take a course for free.

- Practice saying no to anything that doesn't benefit you or your loved one. The world will survive, I promise.

- Write down affirmations or positive statements about yourself. Use note cards or sticky notes so you can keep one on your mirror, one in the car, and one in the kitchen. Seeing them daily helps get their truth into your heart and mind. Rely on these to disrupt negative self-talk.

- Lean on other caregivers to tell you how you're doing with your care. Any noncaregiver's negative opinion belongs in the compost pile with the rest of the manure.

- Get some rest. If you're having trouble sleeping, talk with your doctor. If your loved one is up and down all night, look for family or friends who might sleep over on occasion and run interference. Or hire someone to provide this vital care for you.

- Plan something to look forward to—a trip, a concert, lunch with a friend. Try to always have something you can anticipate with pleasure.

- Expect there to be times when you wish your loved one would die sooner rather than later. Feeling that way doesn't mean you don't love them or that you wish them any harm. It just means you're ready for an end to their suffering and yours.

- Plan for regular breaks from caregiving. These breaks may be short, once or twice a week, or a week that your loved one spends in memory care. If you wait for everyone to be happy about your being away, you'll never go anywhere.

- Spend time on your spiritual life in ways that are meaningful to you. Our souls can get beat up pretty badly with dementia caregiving. Go out of your way to replenish and nourish your spirit.

WHAT TO ASK YOURSELF

Write out your answers to these questions. Save your answers. Revisit the questions once or twice a year. Compare your responses then and now.

- Why did I become a caregiver? (Some say that when you feel like quitting, remember why you began. Be specific in your answers. List at least five reasons. You can do it.)

- What do I value most about myself?

- The best thing I did for my family today was . . .

- The best thing I did for myself today was . . .

- What is it about me that makes my loved one lucky to have me as their caregiver? (Stop worrying about tooting your own horn and answer the question.)

- What have been my greatest successes up to now?

- What is it that I love to do? How can I incorporate that into my days?

- What would I like to learn?

- What am I looking forward to right now? (If the answer is *nothing*, it's time to make a change.)

- What can I do this week/month/year to be kinder to myself?

How Are You Doing?

Taking care of ourselves is something we know we need to do, in theory, at least. In the whirl of a loved one's medical needs, running a household, and possibly working outside the home, it's easy to forget.

When others advise us to get more sleep, eat less junk, or take time out for ourselves, it can feel about as doable as flying to the moon by lunchtime. Like everything else in dementia caregiving, our only hope is to take small steps, one at a time.

Here's a small step you can take this week. Go to the Resources section of this book; under Relaxation Resources (page 162), you'll find the website for a list of meditation apps you can download on your phone. There are various types and durations of meditations. You'll be able to find one to try that suits you.

Download the app to your phone or computer, print the instructions, or follow a video, and commit to spending five minutes a day for the next week trying out a guided meditation. These short, portable meditations can be just the thing to calm your weary mind and reconnect with yourself.

Resources

Be sure to also consult the References section (page 164) for additional sources of information.

GENERAL CAREGIVING ADVICE

- Alzheimer's Reading Room: Award-winning library of practical tips by a former caregiver on hundreds of topics: www.alzheimersreadingroom.com
- *Brain & Life*: Bimonthly magazine with the tagline "Neurology for Everyday Living": www.brainandlife.org
- Better Health While Aging: Consumer information and advice from a geriatric physician: https://betterhealthwhileaging.net
- DailyCaring.com, NextAvenue.org, Caregiver.org, and AgingCare.com: General advice on many dementia caregiving topics
- Advice to share with visitors in advance: https://dailycaring.com /visiting-someone-with-alzheimers-dos-and-donts-for-visitors/

NATIONAL ASSOCIATIONS

- Alzheimer's Association: https://alz.org
- The Association for Frontotemporal Degeneration: www.theaftd.org
- Dementia Friendly America: A clearinghouse for initiatives throughout the United States: www.dfamerica.org/resources
- Lewy Body Dementia Association: www.lbda.org
- TrialMatch (a service of the Alzheimer's Association with information on available clinical trials): https://www.alz.org /alzheimers-dementia/research_progress/clinical-trials /about-clinical-trials

SAFETY RESOURCES

- Alzheimer's Association's Home Safety Checklist: www.alz.org /media/Documents/alzheimers-dementia-home-safety -checklist-ts.pdf
- Alerta: A GPS patch that is applied similar to a medication patch for those who can't or won't wear a bracelet or other hardware: https://trackpatch.com/
- Bedsore Rescue Cushion: Keeps bedridden loved ones positioned to avoid pressure sores and eliminates stuffing pillows or uncomfortable foam wedges: https://bedsorerescue.com/
- How to dementia-proof your home: www.care.com/c/stories /15799/adult-proof-home-dementia/
- Location devices for wanderers: www.alzheimers.net/8-8-14 -location-devices-dementia

FINANCIAL AND LEGAL PLANNING OVERVIEW

- A comprehensive guide from the Alzheimer's Association: www.alz.org/help-support/caregiving/financial-legal-planning

FINANCIAL RESOURCES

- Association for Financial Counseling & Planning Education: www.afcpe.org
- Genworth: Lets you calculate daily, monthly, and annual costs of care in your area: www.genworth.com/aging-and-you/finances /cost-of-care.html
- Where to find free tax preparation help: www.aarp.org/money /taxes/info-2018/aarp-tax-help-fd.html

LEGAL RESOURCES

- An easy-to-use form to help set up an advance directive: https://dementia-directive.org
- Find a Lawyer tool from the National Academy of Elder Law Attorneys: www.naela.org/findlawyer
- Legal advice for those with limited income: www.lawhelp.org

GOVERNMENT BENEFITS

- Aid and Attendance benefits for veterans: www.benefits.va.gov /pension/aid_attendance_housebound.asp
- BenefitsCheckUp: A resource from the National Council on Aging to help you find out what federal, state, and local benefit programs are available in your area: www.benefitscheckup.org
- Medicaid eligibility for long-term care by state: www.seniorplanning.org/long-term-care-medicaid-eligibility/

CHOOSING A LONG-TERM CARE PROVIDER

- Checklist and tips on finding an assisted-living facility: https://dailycaring.com/this-checklist-helps-you-choose-the -right-senior-living-facility/
- Medicare's Hospice Compare tool: www.medicare.gov /hospicecompare
- National Association for Home Care and Hospice: www.nahc.org /consumers-information/home-care-hospice-basics/right-home -care-provider/
- The National Consumer Voice for Quality Long-Term Care: https://theconsumervoice.org/uploads/files/issues /2._How_to_Select_an_Assisted-Living_Facility.pdf

RELAXATION RESOURCES

- Body scanning: www.mindful.org/the-body-scan-practice/
- Meditation apps: https://dailycaring.com/caregivers-get -speedy-meditation-benefits-with-5-simple-apps/
- Mindfulness-based stress reduction, free course: https://palousemindfulness.com/
- Yoga for caregivers: https://blog.ioaging.org/caregiving /yoga-caregivers-poses-affirmations-refresh-empower/

SUPPORT GROUPS

- The Alzheimer's and Dementia Caregivers Support Group (author's online group): www.facebook.com/groups/1661835794070386/
- Emotional support groups for Alzheimer's caregivers: www.alzheimers.net/best-alzheimers-support-groups/
- Memory Cafe Directory: www.memorycafedirectory.com/
- Support groups for caregivers on Facebook: https://dailycaring.com/support-groups-for-caregivers-on-facebook/
- Where to find face-to-face support groups: www.alz.org/events/event_search?etid=2&cid=0

References

AARP. "Caregiving While Working." October 16, 2012. https://www.aarp.
org/caregiving/life-balance/info-2017/work-benefits-rights.html.

Alzheimer's Association. "Anxiety and Agitation." Accessed August 17,
2019. https://www.alz.org/help-support/caregiving/stages-behaviors
/anxiety-agitation.

Alzheimer's Association. "Depression." Accessed August 19, 2019.
https://www.alz.org/help-support/caregiving/stages-behaviors
/depression.

Alzheimer's Association. "Money Matters: Making Financial Plans after a
Diagnosis of Dementia." Accessed September 1, 2019. https://
www.alz.org/national/documents/brochure_moneymatters.pdf.

Alzheimer's Association. "Sleep Issues and Sundowning." Accessed
August 19, 2019. https://www.alz.org/help-support/caregiving
/stages-behaviors/sleep-issues-sundowning.

Alzheimer's Association. "Wandering." Accessed August 19, 2019.
https://www.alz.org/help-support/caregiving/stages-behaviors
/wandering.

Alzheimer's Society. "Depression and Anxiety: Tips for Carers."
Accessed August 19, 2019. https://www.alzheimers.org.uk/about
-dementia/symptoms-and-diagnosis/depression-anxiety-tips
-carers#content-start.

American Geriatrics Society Ethics Committee and Clinical Practice
and Models of Care Committee. "American Geriatrics Society
Feeding Tubes in Advanced Dementia Position Statement." *Journal
of the American Geriatrics Society* 62, no. 8 (August 2014): 1590–93.
doi:10.1111/jgs.12924.

Blair, Brandi. "5 Mistakes I Made with Hired Home Care for My Elderly Parent." *A Bridge between the Gap*. Accessed September 5, 2019. https://abridgebetweenthegap.com/mistakes-with-hired-home-care/.

Creating Daily Joys (blog). "5 Step Hygiene Routine for the Elderly (and Easy on the Caregiver)." July 5, 2015. https://www.creatingdailyjoys .com/5-step-hygiene-for-elderly-easy-for-caregiver/.

Cripe, Brad, Katrina L. Mantzke, and Christopher Bowen. "In-Home Caregivers: Answers to Tax and Nontax Questions." *Journal of Accountancy*. September 1, 2016. https://www.journalofaccountancy. com/issues/2016/sep/taxes-for-caregivers.html.

DailyCaring Editorial Team. "Therapeutic Fibbing: Why Experts Recommend Lying to Someone with Dementia." Accessed September 2019. https://dailycaring.com/why-experts-recommend -lying-to-someone-with-dementia/.

DeMarco, Bob. "7 Ways to Cope with Dementia Patients Who Are Aggressive, Angry or Mean." *Alzheimer's Reading Room*. July 8, 2018. https://www.alzheimersreadingroom.com/2016/06/alzheimer-de-mentia-care-7-ways-to-cope-with-dementia-patients.html.

Dunne, Tracy E., Sandy A. Neargarder, Patsy B. Cipolloni, and Alice Cronin-Golomb. "Visual Contrast Enhances Food and Liquid Intake in Advanced Alzheimer's Disease." *Clinical Nutrition* 23, no. 4 (August 2004): 533–58.

Family Caregiver Alliance. "Work and Eldercare." Accessed September 12 2019. https://www.caregiver.org/work-and-eldercare.

Gaster, Barak, Eric B. Larson, and J. Randall Curtis. "Advance Directives for Dementia." *JAMA* 318, no. 22 (2017): 2175–76. doi:10.1001 /jama.2017.16473.

Gaugler, Joseph E., Eric Jutkowitz, Colleen M. Peterson, and Rachel Zmora. "Caregivers Dying before Care Recipients with Dementia." *Alzheimer's & Dementia: Translational Research & Clinical Interventions* 4 (2018): 688–93. doi:10.1016/j.trci.2018.08.010.

Graff-Radford, Jonathan. "Sundowning: Late-Day Confusion." *Mayo Clinic*. Accessed August 19, 2019. https://www.mayoclinic.org /diseases-conditions/alzheimers-disease/expert-answers /sundowning/faq-20058511.

HealthCentral. "Caregiver Burnout: A Pervasive Problem." October 10, 2018. https://www.healthcentral.com/article/dealing-with -caregiver-burnout?fbclid=IwAR2zhV0pyXvM9zF_0qo4eCmG5.

Help for Alzheimer's Families. "How to Respond to Confusion." Accessed August 19, 2019. https://www.helpforalzheimersfamilies. com/learn/quick-tips/confusion-and-memory-loss/how-to-respond-when-your-loved-one-with-alzheimers-is-confused/.

Hipp, Deb. "What Caregivers Need to Know about FMLA." *A Place for Mom*. September 18, 2017. https://www.aplaceformom.com /blog/what-caregivers-need-to-know-about-fmla/.

Hyatt, Meg. "How to Plan the Legal and Financial Needs of a Loved One with Dementia." *National Elder Law Foundation*. March 1, 2019. https://nelf.org/news/440289/How-To-Plan-The-Legal-And-Financial-Needs-Of-A-Loved-One-With-Dementia.htm.

Kernisan, Leslie. "5 Types of Medication Used to Treat Difficult Alzheimer's Behaviors." *Better Health While Aging*. Accessed August 17, 2019. https://betterhealthwhileaging.net/medications-to-treat-difficult-alzheimers-behaviors/.

Kim, Luke, and Ronan M. Factora. "Alzheimer Dementia: Starting, Stopping Drug Therapy." *Cleveland Clinic Journal of Medicine* 85, no 3 (March 2018): 209–14.

Kirby, Carrie. "12 Questions to Ask When Choosing an Assisted Living Facility." *Wise Bread*. November 1, 2017. https://www.wisebread .com/12-questions-to-ask-when-choosing-an-assisted-living-facility.

Kwak, Yong Tae, YoungSoon Yang, and Min-Seong Koo. "Anxiety in Dementia." *Dementia and Neurocognitive Disorders* 16, no. 2 (2017): 33–39. doi:10.12779/dnd.2017.16.2.33.

Lindau, Stacy T., William Dale, Gillian Feldmeth, Natalia Gavrilova, Kenneth M. Langa, Jennifer A. Makelarski, and Kristen Wroblewski. "Sexuality and Cognitive Status: A U.S. Nationally Representative Study of Home-Dwelling Older Adults." *Journal of the American Geriatrics Society* 66, no. 10 (2018): 1902–10. doi:10.1111/jgs.15511.

Mace, Nancy L. 1984. "Facets of Dementia: Catastrophic Reactions." *Journal of Gerontological Nursing* 10, no. 1 (1984): 38. doi:10.3928 /0098-9134-19840101-08.

Mayo Clinic Staff. "Alzheimer's: Understand Wandering and How to Address It." Accessed August 19, 2019. https://www.mayoclinic.org /healthy-lifestyle/caregivers/in-depth/alzheimers/art-20046222.

Mayo Clinic Staff. "Stress Symptoms: Effects on Your Body and Behavior." Accessed September 10, 2019. https://www.mayoclinic.org /healthy-lifestyle/stress-management/in-depth/stress-symptoms /art-20050987.

Medicaid.gov. "Spousal Impoverishment." Accessed September 3, 2019. https://www.medicaid.gov/medicaid/eligibility/spousal -impoverishment/index.html.

Menzel, Paul T. "Ethical Perspectives on Advance Directives for Dementia." *The Hastings Center*. September 6, 2018. https://www.thehastingscenter.org/ethical-perspectives-advance -directives-dementia/.

Mirelman, Anat, Shirley Shema, Inbal Maidan, and Jeffery M. Hausdorff. "Gait." In *Balance, Gait, and Falls*, edited by Brian L. Day and Stephen R. Lord, *Handbook of Clinical Neurology* 159, 119–34. Amsterdam: Elsevier, 2018.

Orange, Cynthia. "How to Cope with Anticipatory Grief and Ambiguous Loss." *Next Avenue*. September 14, 2017. https://www.nextavenue.org /anticipatory-grief-ambiguous-loss/.

Peck, Kerry R. "Creating Effective Agreements for Payment of Family Caregivers." *ABA*. October 15, 2018. https://www.americanbar

.org/groups/law_aging/publications/bifocal/vol_37/issue
_3_february2016/creating-effective-caregiver-agreements/.

Rackner, Vicki. "Eight Tips to Managing Caregiver Guilt."
Today's Caregiver. Accessed September 11, 2019. https://caregiver.
com/articles/managing_caregiver_guilt/.

Rajan, Vic. "UTIs and Dementia in Seniors: Impact and Treatment
Options." *Aging Care.* Last modified July 25, 2019. https://www.
agingcare.com/articles/urinary-tract-infection-dementia
-in-seniors-155344.htm.

Shabo, Vicki. "Advances in Workplace Protections for Family
Caregivers." *American Society on Aging.* Accessed September 12,
2019. https://www.asaging.org/blog/advances-workplace-protections
-family-caregivers.

UCLA Alzheimer's and Dementia Care Program. "Agitation and
Anxiety." *UCLA Health.* Accessed August 17, 2019.
https://www.uclahealth.org/dementia/agitation-anxiety.

Index

A

Acute medical problems, 5
Adult day care, 100, 102–103, 106
Advance directives, 112–113
Aggression, 36–41
Aging, 5–6
Agitation, 41–44
Alzheimer's disease (AD), 5–6, 8–9, 49
Americans with Disabilities Act
    (ADA), 139
Anger, 36–41
    in caregivers, 128
Antipsychotic drugs, 37–38
Anxiety, 41–44
    in caregivers, 127

B

Bathing, 76–80
Body scanning, 134
Brain failure, 4

C

Caregiving. *See also* Self-care
    arranging outside services, 141–142
    balancing work with, 138–140
    emotional and physical tolls of,
        126–131
    grief and loss, 131–133
Care teams, 26–29
Catastrophic reactions, 37
Certified nursing assistants (CNA), 99
Clergy, 27
Clinical trials, 28
Cognition, 4
Confusion, 47–50
Consent, 84–85
Counselors, 27
Creutzfeldt-Jakob Disease, 13

D

Delirium, 5–6
Dementia
    defined, 3–4
    diagnosis, 16–18
    symptoms, 6–7
    types, 7–16
Depression, 45–47
    in caregivers, 128–129
Diagnostic procedures, 16–18
Dining out, 66–67
Doctors, 18, 26, 31
Driving, 81–83

E

Eating, 64–67
Elder law attorneys, 95
End-of-life decisions, 112–116
Exercise, 146–148
Exhaustion, 130

F

Family and Medical Leave Act
    (FMLA), 138–139
Feeding tubes, 65, 113
Fiblets, 56
Finances, 90–94
Frontotemporal dementia, 11–12
Frustration, 128
Full-time facility care, 100–101, 103–
    104, 106–107

G

Geriatric psychiatrists, 26, 38
Grief, 131–133
Guardianship, 95
Guilt, 129–130

H

Home health care, 99, 102–103, 105–106
Home safety, 80–83
Hospice care, 116–119
Huntington's Disease (HD), 14
Hydration, 64–65

I

Incontinence, 67–70
Intimacy, 23, 83–86

L

Legal matters, 30, 94–98
Lewy body dementia (LBD), 10–11
Living wills, 112–113
Long-term care, 98–108
Loss, 131–133

M

Medical centers, 28
Medical power of attorney, 112–113
Medications, 30, 37–38, 49
  administering, 70–73
Memory cafés, 153
Memory care centers, 100–101, 103–104,
  106–107
Memory loss, 47–51
Mild cognitive impairment (MCI), 5
Mindfulness-based stress reduction
  (MBSR), 45–46
Mixed dementia, 11
Mobility, 73–76

N

Neurologists, 26
Normal pressure hydrocephalus
  (NPH), 13–14
Nurses, 27
Nutrition, 64–67

O

Occupational therapists, 27, 74

P

Parkinson's disease dementia, 12–13
Personal hygiene, 76–80
Physical therapists, 27, 74
Pick's disease, 12
Posterior cortical atrophy (PCA), 15–16
Power of attorney documents, 92, 95, 112–113
Psychotherapists, 27

R

Record-keeping, 29–31
Relationships, 22–26, 31–32
Repetitive actions, 50–53
Restaurants, 66–67

S

Sadness, 128–129
Safety, 80–83
Self-care
  actions, 18–19, 31–32, 59–60, 86–87,
    108, 120, 134, 143, 158
  connecting with friends and family,
    150–152
  diet and nutrition, 148–149
  exercise, 146–148
  self-kindness, 155–158
  support groups, 87, 127, 152–154
Sex, 23, 83–86
Social workers, 27
Spiritual advisors, 27
Stress, 127
Sundowning, 53–55
Support groups, 87, 127, 152–154

T

Therapists, 27

V

Vascular dementia, 9–10

W

Walking, 73–76
Wandering, 55–59
Wernicke-Korsakoff syndrome
  (WKS), 15

Acknowledgments

This book has lived in my head and heart for many years. Bits and pieces would leak out onto the page and then stall.

Over the years, my book dreams were sustained by the friends who believed in me relentlessly until I could believe in myself: Beth Valorz and family plus all my Life Group soul mates, especially Darlene Groome and Mike Drew.

I thank the team at Callisto Media for holding my feet to the fire to finally get the book out of my head and into the world. Seth Schwartz, my editor, has my lifelong gratitude.

Many thanks to mentor Catie Harris, RN, PhD, and to Anne Marie Labenberg, RN, MSN, who reviewed my work through an expert nurse's eyes.

Finally, with a humble heart, I thank my number one cheer-leaders, the amazing whirlwinds of stardust, sass, and love that I call daughters, Katie Danielle and Bonnie Anne Weatherill.

About the Author

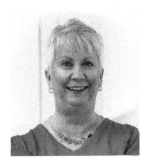

Gail Weatherill has been a registered nurse for 40 years. For the past two decades, she has specialized in the care of people living with dementia and their families. A former director of nursing in long-term care, Gail is a certified Alzheimer's educator and now trains and coaches family and professional caregivers as "the Dementia Nurse."

Gail is the cofounder of the Alzheimer's and Dementia Caregivers Support Group, a closed Facebook group that now serves 50,000 members from more than 100 countries. She has written on nursing care of families in crisis, symptom control at the end of life, alternative therapies in dementia care, and the failure of medical and faith communities in supporting people with dementia.

A past recipient of the American Association of Critical-Care Nurses' Excellence in Caring Practices Award, Gail is a longtime resident of Charlottesville, Virginia. An alumna of the University of Virginia, she is a rabid fan of UVA sports and a spoiled-rotten Maine coon cat named Baby Silas. You can learn more about Gail's advocacy at www.TheDementiaNurse.com.

Printed in the USA
CPSIA information can be obtained
at www.ICGtesting.com
LVHW051919170124
769161LV00056B/2482